LIVE WELL, SLEEP WELL

LIVE WELL, SLEEP WELL

The Holistic Way to a Good Night's Sleep

Dan Campbell

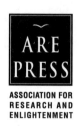

ARE PRESS

**ASSOCIATION FOR
RESEARCH AND
ENLIGHTENMENT**

A.R.E. Press • Virginia Beach • Virginia

A.R.E. Press
215 67th Street
Virginia Beach, VA 23451-2061

Campbell, Dan.
    Live well, sleep well : the holistic way to a good night's sleep
/ by Dan Campbell.
        p.   cm.
Includes bibliographical references.
ISBN 0-87604-426-7
    1. Sleep. 2. Holistic medicine. 3. Cayce, Edgar, 1877-1945.
Edgar Cayce readings. I. Title.
RA786.C36   2000
613.7'9—dc21

                                00-058300

A Note to the Reader:

No part of this book is intended to substitute for competent medical
diagnosis, nor does the A.R.E. endorse any of the information contained herein as prescription for the treatment of disease. Edgar Cayce
gave health readings for particular individuals with specific conditions; therefore, any application of his advice in present-day diet
planning should be undertaken only after consulting with a certified
nutrition expert or other professional practitioner in a related field. It
is especially important that you do not discontinue any prescribed
diet or treatment without the full concurrence of your doctor.

Grateful acknowledgment is made to the following for reprint per-
mission:
George G. Ritchie, M.D., for *Return from Tomorrow,* Chosen Books,
    Waco, Texas, 1978.
Deepak Chopra, M.D., for *Ageless Body, timeless Mind: The Quantum
    Alternative to Growing Old,* Harmony Books, 1993.

Cover design by Lightbourne

Dedication

This book is for my daughter, Robin,
who once asked me to write something for her.

Contents

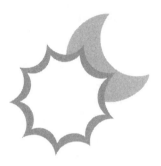

FOREWORD

Several summers ago, Hurricane Bonnie crippled my Virginia Beach neighborhood. Fortunately, no one was injured by uprooted trees or falling limbs, but the wind played havoc with the power lines. We weren't surprised when the lights went out—they often do during summer squalls here at the beach. As nightfall approached, we scurried about the house, lighting candles, and rather enjoyed the romantic atmosphere they created from room to room. By the next day, however, we began to fret over the contents of our immobilized refrigerator and to feel uncomfortable without air conditioning. And without television or radio, we weren't sure how badly Bonnie had treated us or how long before we could expect restoration of our modern conveniences.

By the second night of darkness, we realized that there

was little we could do once the daylight faded out. I tried finishing a novel by candlelight, but gave up when I realized that my wife was right when she cautioned me about hurting my eyes. So, we went to bed and slept until dawn's early light allowed us to start another round of activities. Instead of being annoyed by our deprived circumstances, however, we talked about how this was the way it was for the human race for much of our history on the planet, working dawn to dusk, sleeping through the dark hours.

For three days, we experienced life without artificial light or mechanical noise (except for distant chain saws clearing the roads of tree trunks), and life seemed more mellow, relaxed, and conducive to rest than our normally noisy routine, which pushed us to the limits of exhaustion. Even though it was warm and humid without our cooling system, we slept longer than usual. Insomnia, I ventured, was not a problem for our ancestors. It was my first insight into why a good night's sleep is harder to come by today.

A friend who has a sleep disorder for which he takes a prescribed medication recalls that when he lived in a monastery, as a Roman Catholic priest, he never had trouble sleeping. When I asked what hours they kept, he described the routine much as I had experienced it during our blackout: The priests turned in at 8:30 p.m. and arose for morning prayers at 4:30 a.m. My guess is that this dawn-to-dusk schedule was as old as their religion.

Dan Campbell traces the beginnings of our trouble with sleeping to Edison's most successful invention, the light bulb; and after my "lights out" encounter with Bonnie, I think he has got it right. It is ironic that Edison would probably never accept the blame, since he thought we didn't really need to devote all that much time to sleeping. The evidence from health authorities is otherwise.

Given the utility of electricity for brightening our lives in so many ways, there is no turning back the clock. But there are ways of getting the rest that our health requires, if we wisely guard against the disturbing influences we can control.

As in so many areas of life, we really need to assume responsibility for the outcome and know that we can have what we need without compromising our health or retreating from contemporary life. Dan Campbell leads us through the temptations of the quick fix to a better solution for taking control and dealing creatively with our physical, mental, and spiritual needs for adequate rest.

Read it, and sleep well.

A. Robert Smith
*Misdiagnosed: Was My Wife a Casualty
of America's Medical Cold War?*

PREFACE

When the publisher of *Live Well, Sleep Well* and I first discussed the idea of a book that delves into sleep and insomnia, my first thought was whether these subjects had already received ample attention for the time being. A number of books dealing with sleep and sleep disorders had appeared during the past decade alone. Exactly what could another book offer to justify its existence?

The answer to this question is in your hands. Initially, after several weeks of reviewing numerous publications, I discovered a puzzling fact: Of the many books about sleep and sleep disorders, only one modest volume even came close to treating the subject holistically; that is, from a body-mind perspective. This book, however, completes the holistic connection in that it includes consideration of the spiritual. The spiritual dimension of our beings, as you will discover, is reckoned by our inner states, and plays an especially active and influential role during sleep.

In pursuit of investigating the subject of sleep from a holistic viewpoint, I have relied on information gleaned from the psychic discourses of Edgar Cayce, who provided clairvoyant guidance for many thousands of people on numerous topics for half a century. The range of Cayce's mind while in a trance state reached well beyond the boundaries of the sensory world to which science is necessarily limited. While researchers are not altogether certain about what sleep is, the psychic readings provide fascinating clarification of this nocturnal activity and its bearing on the human condition. Cayce looked at body, mind, and soul as facets of one nature; thus, his advice and recommendations to others were based on a holistic premise. I believe you will find the insights and suggestions presented here as engaging and helpful as I did while assembling this material.

My gratitude is extended to editors Brenda English, Ruth O'Lill, and Bob Smith for their insights and suggestions. Sincere thanks also goes to the considerate and patient staff of the A.R.E. Library; and a special note of appreciation is due Joan C. Beggs of the Wal-Mart pharmacy chain for providing explanatory data regarding various medications discussed in these pages.

This Thing Called Sleep

If only one thing might be said about the twentieth century, it is that it was a very busy 100 years. Even without the distractions of two world wars and countless other wars and conflicts, it was a period of unprecedented expansion and activity in pursuit of innovation and development. Except for an economic pothole in the century's road called the Great Depression, everything seemed to mushroom, including the population. Technological advances were continually served up like an endless smorgasbord from which increasing numbers of consumers could feast to satisfy their needs for goods and services.

Modern conveniences were designed for comfort, efficiency, and, when applicable, speed. Speed above all. As the century rolled on at an ever faster pace and provided us with more choices, our appetite for diversion and entertainment increased. One invention in particular bought us more time to indulge our leisure: incandescent light. The hours of the day were extended to well after dark. Compared with the relatively lackluster illumination from kerosene and gas lamps, electric light was a dazzling improvement. It may well be that no other device has affected our lives more personally. Although a late nineteenth-century accomplishment, the electric light helped changed the civilized world within a few short decades. For instance, the first night baseball game was played in 1935. We were given more and more reasons to stay up longer in the evenings. But as the light spread across the landscape and illuminated our world, there was also an increase in a peculiar ailment: insomnia. Sleeplessness was the price of progress.

Three decades ago, physiotherapist Harold J. Reilly surveyed modern life and expressed his conclusion in *The Edgar Cayce Handbook for Health Through Drugless Therapy*. His view appears even truer today:

Millions of people in the so-called civilized world are suffering from "future shock." The last half-century has tremendously increased the speed, quantity, and range of sensory stimuli that strike the brain. Our senses of sight, hearing, smell, taste, and touch are assaulted by man-made pollution at every waking and sleeping moment. The increase of tension in modern life—the competitive strains in work, worry, and insecurity all adding up to stresses, and even in so-called recreation and leisure—are being discussed ad nauseam with appropriate alarm in all the media, and fill the psychiatrists' offices with patients. The consequences can be observed in the increase in mental disease, drug addiction, and alcoholism, and in a population of pill-poppers living on tranquilizers, stimulants, and sleeping pills, swallowed like candy in the search for peace of mind and soul.

Progress has come at a price, and one of the ways we pay for our progress is with loss of sleep. At the same time, it is somehow fitting that the man who invented the incandescent lightbulb, Thomas Edison, believed sleep was unnecessary. Edison was a technological genius, and his inventions are legion, the motion picture projector and phonograph among them. It was almost as if he could devise whatever he dreamed up and give utilitarian form to his visions. There is also irony in the thought that dreams played no role that we know of in Edison's 1,000-plus patented inventions. It is not at all unusual for inventors, and others, to receive guidance through sleep by dreaming of solutions to difficult problems. A famous case in point was Elias Howe's dream of being attacked by African tribesmen wielding spears with holes in the tips. This dream image provided him with the answer that made the sewing machine an efficient device.

But it may be that Edison had no dream life to speak of, perhaps because he logged no more than about four hours of sleep a night. He not only deemed sleep unnecessary, he also held a certain disdain for it and believed that the hours in an unconscious state held back progress, using up productive time and making people stupid and lazy. We can only imagine what kind of response he might have received if he had voiced his opinion to a mob of grouchy insomniacs. At any rate, Edison also believed that in time sleep would be eradicated altogether once people had sufficient illumination. His invention, incandescent light, certainly changed our work and sleep habits when the wheels of work and play continued rolling through the late hours as the light turned night into day.

Being the practical and self-promoting soul that he was, Edison could only presume that if a few hours of sleep were adequate for his needs, then that should be enough for everyone. If only he could see us now, a country in which, according to the estimates of some experts, as many as fifty million people suffer from insomnia and other sleep disorders, he might reconsider his conclusion. The per capita number of sufferers is likely the same in other industrial countries. It is a pandemic of sleep deprivation. While insomnia may be as old as creation—beginning at about the time Adam and Eve vacated the Garden of Eden's premises—it appears to be more of a modern ailment, the piper who is being paid for our modern progress, judging by the startling number of sufferers today. Treating sleep disorders has grown into a virtual industry. The American Academy of Sleep Medicine counts about 3,400 individual members and 300 member sleep disorders centers. Almost all the states in the U.S. have sleep centers dedicated to treating the increasing numbers of people suffering from sleep disorders.

Contrary to Edison's prescription, the need for many people is not to eliminate sleep, but to get enough quality sleep and to get it regularly. If you are one of those who suffer from a sleep deficiency, you are well aware of the toll insufficient sleep takes on your efficiency and production on the job, your social life and relationships, your state of mind, and your well-being.

There is no doubt that sleep wields a powerful control that even our wills cannot nullify beyond a certain point. To push the envelope of wakefulness to the extent that sleep occurs almost unexpectedly can have tragic consequences. Anyone who has nodded off for a second or two while driving realizes the dangers of suddenly falling asleep. Some people, unfortunately, lose consciousness at the wheel and never wake up again. It is estimated that 100,000 automobile accidents are caused annually by drivers falling asleep at the wheel.

What is sleep? Scientists still can't say for sure. Even after decades of investigating sleep processes, researchers are able to describe only what happens biologically within body and brain. It was once thought that sleep is a kind of suspended animation, but this turns out to be an accurate analogy. The metabolism of the body, for instance, slows down only about ten percent during sleep, while the brain remains active, moving in and out of various stages of slumber. Instead of shutting down, the brain undergoes a shift in consciousness.

Just why we need to sleep isn't altogether clear to scientists, despite years of research. There is no consensus among experts, only speculation, as to why we need daily periods of unconsciousness. There are people who obviously get by quite well on less than the recommended norm of eight hours' sleep, indicating it is an individual matter that possibly relates to lifestyle, habits, and the amount of stress with which one has to deal. That some people need less sleep than others—in many instances considerably less—also suggests that it is not merely the number of hours spent in slumber that is important, but also the quality of the rest afforded the body and the mind.

What is known for sure is that sleep is wired to the body's biologic clock, to our circadian cycles as a necessary break in our daily routines. When we are deprived of sufficient sleep, it is also certain that life can be hell. But how necessary is sleep? Experiments have shown that persons deprived of sleep for a night or two can still effectively carry out complicated tasks. Some people perform relatively well even after several days of sleeplessness. It has been found, however, that experimental subjects who remained awake for extended periods while their brain-wave patterns were monitored would nod off, if only for seconds and even with their eyes taped open. Obviously when the body needs sleep, it will grab any it can get, even fleeting snatches lasting only a moment.

Occasional loss of sleep has little ill effect if you make up some of the loss. It is not necessary to recoup the exact amount of loss to catch up. If you miss two hours' sleep one night, for instance, going to bed an hour earlier than usual the following evening or sleeping later may settle the deficit. Even a greater loss might be made up with only an extra hour or two. Just how much time is required to balance the books, of course, probably depends on the quality of your slumber in general.

It is helpful to keep in mind that if you suffer from chronic insomnia, getting the night's sleep you need, and getting it regularly, are not likely to be achieved with one remedy. A number of adjustments may be called for. Repeated sleep loss affects other aspects of your life. A specific disorder may begin with a single change in your routine, such as switching work schedules from the day to night shift, a situation which can set off a kind of domino effect, upsetting your routines and adversely affecting your personal life. Although ongoing bouts of sleeplessness should be considered a symptom of disease (in the Cayce sense of the body being out of balance)—and even a sign of possible illness—frequent loss may also act as a catalyst that can create other disturbances.

Insomnia is a catchall term for the inability to get enough sleep. Broadly, insomnia is the inability to fall asleep for an extended period after retiring or a failure to remain asleep. While the amount of rest needed varies among people, "enough sleep" implies that the sleeper awakens feeling rested and refreshed. The fact that no dregs of fogginess cling to your mind when you wake up, however, does not mean that you are fully revitalized. As you will see, insomnia takes various forms.

Slow to Arrive

You switch off the TV, climb into bed, and turn out the lamp. Or after reading in bed for a while, you lay aside the book or magazine and nestle your head in the pillow. You close your eyes. You lie there. And lie there. A half-hour later, you are still awake. After an hour of sleeplessness, you resume whatever you were doing before you presumed to call it a night, only to repeat the process the next hour.

The inability to fall asleep within a reasonable time is the most common version of insomnia. Its causes may be many, but to lie awake for long stretches before your conscious mind manages to close down for the night is frustrating to say the least. And it is downright irritating when you must rise early the next morning. The difficulty with surrendering to annoyance and frustration is that these are sleep robbers, which make it even more difficult to fall asleep sooner than later. Intense emotions of any kind—whether negative or positive—only compound the problem of falling asleep within a reasonable time after retiring.

Short and Sweet

Another common habit—which happens as we grow older—is to fall asleep within a reasonable time, sleep several hours, then wake up for the duration without feeling sleepy. This may be a sign that you have had adequate shut-eye. If not, the effects will catch up with you later in the day; you will feel fatigued, and your muscles may ache or feel stiff. Some people tend to fret about what they perceive as curtailed sleep because they have accepted the fiction that everyone needs eight hours of sleep a night, every night, all their lives. We may not need as much sleep as we assume. When monitored by researchers, some self-diagnosed insomniacs were found to get more sleep than they thought they received. When sleep is curtailed one night, the problem usually corrects itself the following evening when a full night's rest balances the offset. If brief sleep happens only occasionally, it is no cause for concern.

Shallow and Unsettled

What if you fall asleep readily, but on waking do not feel particularly rested? Then you are a light sleeper, one who floats close to the surface of consciousness most of the night. In fact, you probably surface several times, but you do not recall these momentary periods of waking. If you reach the deepest level of sleep at all, your visits are short. The shallow sleeper is easily disturbed, of course, and if the environment is not conducive to peace and quiet, the quality of relaxation suffers whether the person wakes fully or not.

This is pure speculation, but aside from the inability to fully relax because of external conditions, it might be that a light sleeper is avoiding unpleasant dreams. Some authorities believe this can be the case. Few things corrode the quality of rest as surely as reveries beset by a stormy sea of troubles or infiltrated by nightmares that shock you awake. Disturbing dreams are frequently delivered with vivid images that drive the sleeper back to consciousness in a panic. You may dream of falling or being pushed from the rooftop of a high building, of being chased by someone, of being threatened by a sinister figure holding a gun or knife. A dream doesn't need scary visual effects, however, to undermine sleep. You may be alone in your dream in a kind of void yet feel overwhelmed by a sense of impending but undefinable doom or a vague awareness that something disastrous is about to happen.

Frightening dreams come in many guises. A tableau may appear benign as far as the events themselves are concerned, yet leave us feeling somehow distressed or uneasy. What awakens the dreamer is not what is happening in the nightmare as much as the person's emotional reaction to it. Does this suggest that what we take for granted as illusory—the dream—may be a separate dimension of reality? A separate consciousness? Or are we simply absorbed by the action and images as if watching a movie? Either way, we often make quite an emotional investment in the dream content. It is not waking up that calms our panic so much as having the threat removed when we leave that inner dimension. Yet even then the intense emotional residue—sweating, racing heart, panic—is real. Dreams, of course, don't have to be unpleasant to rouse us. Any kind of electrifying episode can do the trick—from winning a lottery to a sexual scenario.

There are many types of disorders associated with sleep that disturb quality rest. Among these are narcolepsy, night terrors, sleep paralysis, sleepwalking, restless-legs syndrome, bedwetting, and teeth grinding. If you suffer from any of these or other sleep-related disorders, you should consider seeing a physician or sleep therapist for appropriate treatment.

Do You Suffer from Insomnia?

Do you believe you are a chronic insomniac? Keep in mind that everyone goes through an occasional siege of sleeplessness. The loss is usually self-correcting; a short night of rest is followed by a longer one, and a long sleep by a shorter night's rest. Most of us are realistic about our sleep patterns without becoming overly concerned about occasional loses. A common syndrome is for many people to repeat a weekly spate of insomnia-like experiences following weekends during which they have allowed their usual routines to become disrupted by staying up much later than normal. Also, many people are convinced they suffer from insomnia when in fact they get adequate amounts of sleep. According to studies, about half the people who claim they sleep little actually get more sleep than they believe. Pseudo-insomniacs who estimated an hour or so passed before they fell asleep were found slumbering within fifteen minutes after going to bed. Perhaps it is the excessive concern about the importance of performing well during waking hours that causes people to miscalculate the time it takes them to fall asleep.

If you believe you may be developing a chronic insomnia problem, you should take stock of your sleep habits and routine. Review the following questions and, if any occur constantly or on a regular basis, it's time for you to take action by following the suggestions in this book:

Do you:
• Have trouble going to sleep within a reasonable time, even when you feel tired?
• Wake up during the night and can't go back to sleep right away?
• Feel extremely sleepy at times during the day?
• Get sleepy whenever you just sit quietly or while reading or watching TV?
• Fall asleep unintentionally at times?
• Have to force yourself to get out of bed in the morning?
• Have difficulty waking up easily when the alarm clock sounds?
• Oversleep most mornings during the work week?

Although there is a great deal about sleep that we don't know, few states seem as natural to us. We take it for granted—unless, of course, we have difficulty sleeping. At such times sleep can take on the indifference of an alienated friend, and for all its naturalness it is a fascinating fact that sleep cannot be induced at will. It obviously follows the beat of a different drummer. In *Restful Sleep*, Deepak Chopra emphasizes that "Sleep is a natural process, and 'trying' will have no positive effect. Trying will probably aggravate the insomnia."

What *may* have a positive effect is a self-inventory. Many people apparently overlook the value of appraising their lifestyles and habits in connection with difficulty sleeping. It is a cause-and-effect world, of course, and insomnia doesn't just happen for no reason. The causes aren't always apparent, but you hold the answers. Chronic or persistently recurring bouts of insomnia are related to numerous causes, which in many cases are found in the insomniacs themselves. Sleep expert Peter Hauri in his informative book *No More Sleepless Nights* reveals:

> According to national statistics and our own experience, at least half of all insomnias are caused by psychological problems such as depression, anxiety, marital stress, or job stress. (It does *not* mean when we talk about a psychological problem that you are crazy or psychotic, which is very rare in insomniacs.)
>
> We find, however, that the insomniac typically is the very last person to know that his or her problem is associated with psychological issues. Like most people, insomniacs typically do not want to think of themselves as having an emotional or psychological problem. Therefore, even though you do not think your problem is psychological, consider that the chances are at least 50-50 that you might belong in this category. At the clinic, we often find that everybody around the insomniac knew that psychologi-

cal help was needed, though the insomniac was to-
tally unaware of this.

Studies of brain waves have provided some insights
for researchers who study sleep and related disorders. In
the early 1950s it was determined that there are two types
of sleep: rapid-eye-movement (REM) sleep and non-REM
sleep. It was assumed that the darting movements of the
eyes indicate that the sleeper is observing active images
in dreams. Some studies have shown that eye movements
appear to coincide with the motions in dream sequences.
Also, the higher brain functions are quite active during
REM sleep, while muscular movements of the body are
usually restricted, except for facial twitches. There was
once an accepted misconception that the brain remains
inactive or idle during sleep, perhaps because of the notion that, like the body, it needs rest. Yet, to the contrary,
researchers have found that during the REM stage the
brain seems to reach peak activity and may be even more
active than in the waking state. These factors complicate
questions regarding the nature of sleep, thus a definitive
answer remains obscure to investigators.

Specialists have divided sleep into four stages—though
some researchers include REM sleep as the fifth state—
which are based on brain-wave patterns of sleepers as
recorded by an electroencephalograph (EEG). It isn't simply that we go to sleep and then awaken; we shift through
different levels of unconsciousness, passing in and out of
each stage several times during the night. There are
marked distinctions among these stages while intricate
changes occur in the brain and body.

When scientists began attaching EEG electrodes to
sleepers, they soon discovered that the brain remains
surprisingly active, especially during the REM stage.
When you are awake, relaxed, and passive, the EEG will
scribble a pattern revealing that your brain waves are

pulsing along at eight to thirteen cycles per second. In stage-four sleep, the deepest level recorded, the waves are creeping along at one-half to two-and-one-half cycles per second. During REM sleep, the tracings of the brain waves register at thirteen to fifteen cycles per second, equaling the wave patterns of a brain that is very much alert and aware, and hardly passive. Consider the ramifications: The brain is asleep—unconscious—to the objective world, but wide awake in its subjective reality. But more about this in a later chapter.

If Thomas Edison could see us now. He might realize that he jumped to a conclusion not reckoned by reality. He would find a world in which sleep has become a commodity in its own right. Hotels, inns, and resorts everywhere are promoting sleeping accommodations as a main attraction of their facilities. Following suit, mattress manufacturers aren't merely promoting their bedding, but the comfortable, satisfying, and sound sleep it provides for weary bones. And perhaps if Edison had had similar bedding in his day, he might have slept longer.

The last century was indeed busy. The emphasis we gave technology almost defines it as a time dominated by our attention to things. But it also produced more than a few unique individuals, incomparable souls such as Albert Schweitzer, Mohandas Gandhi, Mother Teresa, and Martin Luther King, Jr., as well as numerous stellar personalities who, instead of giving us things, dedicated their lives to improving the human condition and, in the process, quickened our spirits and strengthened our faith. Among many other unique persons, though perhaps lesser known to the population at large, one man dedicated his life to helping others by providing them with information: Edgar Cayce, the psychic and "sleeping prophet." His adult life spanned the first half of the twentieth century, during which he gave clairvoyant readings

"that benefited thousands of people who sought guidance through him.

This information still provides insights into countless
topics, many of which are relevant to the issues discussed
in this book. Some of these psychic insights and discourses—drawn from among more than 14,000 readings—will be included in upcoming chapters because it
is, at times, exceptional information that continues to
benefit the human condition physically, mentally, and
spiritually. For the clairvoyant Cayce, there was no question about the purpose of sleep: It isn't simply a physical
activity alone, as you will discover.

2

The Pace and Rhythm of Our Lives

The changes that occurred during the last century were phenomenal. The electric light may have brightened our nights, but our lives were made easier in numerous other ways. Modern gadgets such as the washing machine simplified daily chores. We began to travel in ways and at speeds unimaginable to our nineteenth-century ancestors. In the annals of recorded time, no century preceding it even came close to its achievements. Yet, while our lives have been made better outwardly, we seem to be paying a heavy toll inwardly. The primary coin of this modern realm is stress. We embrace the newer and better and faster, but at the expense of making our everyday world more hectic; we avidly pursue diversions to avoid boredom, but at the cost of inner peace.

Throughout the eons, the human condition has never

been entirely free of stress, but modern life has added an elaborate mix of causes. Stress, of course, is a prime har-binger of insomnia. In *Everybody's Guide to Sleep*, Philip Goldberg and Daniel Kaufman point out:

> The character of modern life—with its pressures, changes, pollutants, noise, overstimulation, and manifold nuisances—can wreak havoc on the endo-crine and nervous systems, throwing the body's natural rhythms out of balance. The result can be a disruption of your natural sleep rhythms.

These various factors continue churning up a flood of insomniacs and victims of sleep disorders. Stresses come in many forms, though they are not necessarily limited to negative influences. But whether you win the lottery or your pet dies, the impact is stressful. A positive stress, however, may seem more tolerable because it boosts your morale, yet it's still a shock to your nervous system. Like the sleeper's reaction to a dream, it is not merely what is happening but how you react to a sudden change in your life and its effect on you that are the real measure of stressful impact on you.

Yet, this is true only to a point. To explore just one example already mentioned, consider noise. We humans are capable of relaxing and achieving a more or less placid state only when we are not confronted with a threat or challenge—or a teeth-gritting annoyance. Loud noises that go on constantly, for instance, are abrasive to your nervous system even if you are by nature the most serene person in the world. Add up the cacophony of sounds that may bombard your body daily and you get an idea of how you might well end up restless or edgy, even if only slightly, after an otherwise good day. This is no small matter. Noise and sound are vibrations, which are felt by your entire body and not simply the ears alone. In addition, the vibrations need not be audible in order to disturb you. Goldberg and Kaufman point up the case of French factory workers who inexplicably began suffering from fatigue, irritability, and nausea. The mysterious cause of the ailments, as it turned out, were the "sounds" from newly installed machinery—sounds which were undetectable by the human ear, yet nevertheless produced an upsetting effect on the nervous systems of the workers.

Endocrine Glands

Consideration of the endocrine system in connection with stress is important, because this system controls many functions and plays a vital role in the health of the body. In conjunction with the nervous system, it serves as the control center of the body's vitality and immune system. The pituitary, for example, produces several hormones that, among other things, promote muscle and physical growth and play a part in the general metabolism of the body. The endocrine glands are given a great deal of attention throughout the Cayce readings. And from his clairvoyant perspective he was well aware of the interrelationship among the seven glands and how they affect one another. When giving a "physical" reading on a person's health, particularly for a serious or chronic condition, Cayce made it a point to evaluate how well these glands were coordinating their functions. To purify the glands and to aid their operation, he commonly suggested the use of Atomidine, which, as he put it, is iodine with the poisons removed. It was also recommended for numerous other purposes, with the application or the dosage tailored to the condition and the individual.

For example, in reading 2015-8, given in 1941, the parents of a two-year-old girl put this question to Cayce, "What can be done as a precaution to keep her from

contracting Infantile Paralysis [polio] . . . ?" He replied,
"Every other day give one drop of Atomidine in half a
glass of water, before the morning meal. Keep this up for
five days, skip five, and repeat—continuing in this manner through the winter." His recommended dosage for an
adult to prevent the same disease was two drops daily,
five days on and five off. He noted that Atomidine was to
the endocrine system what oil is to a machine. (Use of
Atomidine, of course, should not be undertaken without
a doctor's approval if you are taking other forms of iodine supplements or are being treated for a thyroid condition.)

William McGarey, M.D., who has written and lectured
extensively on the Cayce medical readings, recommends
the following regimen for anyone who wants to use
Atomidine: one drop in a glass of water on Monday and
two on Tuesday, adding a drop each day until five drops
are consumed on Friday. None is taken during the week-
end. Resume the progression on Monday with one drop,
etc. Repeat for three weeks, discontinue for a week, and
then begin again.

Attitudes and Emotions

Your life is chock-full of things that go bump in your
nervous system, producing tension and stress, which, in
turn, wreck your sleep. You may be able to slough off the
usual frustrations of the day, such as those that arise from
traffic snarls or some job-related headache, but enough of
these small ingredients can add up to a restless night in
bed; or toss in an argument with your spouse or boss and
you can kiss sleep goodnight. If you are fortunate, you
will make up the loss the following night and get back on
schedule. In some cases, however, the first episode of
insomnia produces a kind of domino effect, one night
after another of poor sleep, thus turning a molehill of

curtailed sleep into a mountain of habitual loss of shut-eye.

Needless to say, it isn't external circumstances or other people alone that cause you to lose sleep. There are also internal causes, and none is more important than your attitudes and emotions. These are largely byproducts of temperament, your individual nature. Their importance to your well-being cannot be stressed too much. Few things provide a more telling barometer of who and what you are than your attitudes and emotions, which more often than not are reflected in the pace and rhythm of your life, the mark of your lifestyle.

Attitudes and emotions can make or break you. When you are upbeat and positive, you feel cheerful, energetic, buoyant; when downcast and negative, you feel sour, dispirited, burdened. Other descriptions apply, of course, depending on the specific barometric reading of your mood. Keep in mind, too, that the longer you subscribe to a mood, the more ingrained it becomes. Without question, mind is the builder, an idea echoed countless times throughout the readings. When Cayce diagnosed an ailment, his evaluation was not made merely from an organic perspective, but from the molecular and atomic perspectives as well as noting the psychological disposition of the person. He explained in reading 137-81 that every physical being is composed of atomic forces, that each atom is a universe in itself with a mind of its own that is under the supervision and influence of the body's mental faculties. When someone is ill, for instance, "all the attributes of the mind . . . become then paramount" in furnishing the impetus within the body to bring about healing conditions. When healing occurs for no discernible reason, it is sometimes explained away as the "placebo effect," though we are assured by the readings that the thoughts and attitudes of the person are major contributors to overcoming an illness. As Norman Cousins observed in *Anatomy of an Illness*, "The placebo is the doctor who resides within."

Attitudes and emotions directly affect your nervous and endocrine systems, and as reading 294-208 explains, the secretions of the glands take their cue from your emotions. If you consider these secretions on an atomic level, you understand why it is important to maintain a proper state of mind at all costs, because your thoughts, which fuel your moods, can affect the nature of these secretions, which in turn can have a healthy influence on the body or undermine its well-being, thus resulting in illness as well as inhibiting the healing process. This cause-and-effect principle between mind and body is emphasized plainly in reading 4021-1: "No one can hate his neighbor and not have stomach or liver trouble. No one can be jealous and allow the anger of same [to eat at him] and not have upset digestion or heart disorder."

Psychologist Peter Alimaras identifies "cognitive distortions" as the source of certain emotional patterns. These distortions include various types of destructive thinking such as over-generalization, jumping to conclusions, and all-or-none thinking, Alimaras reports in *How to Change Your Mind*. Many psychological problems are accompanied by anger, sadness, and nervousness, which can become ingrained when the validity of the thought patterns behind our emotions goes unquestioned. Alimaras emphasizes, "The important thing . . . is that the emotion relates to the way the situation is interpreted." Or to put it another way, our interpretations of circumstances define how we feel. Also, it might be added that our interpretations/feelings establish our personal reality.

When we view our emotions in a more objective light, a peculiar fact becomes evident: We tend to take it for granted that the way we feel, the way we react to circumstances, is "just the way we are." This is particularly the case when it comes to negative emotions. Ill-natured feelings burrow quickly within and hang on like parasites. Positive feelings and moods seem somehow ephemeral in comparison. The reason may be that emotions are coping mechanisms, as some experts believe, that help relieve stress. Negative emotions are particularly those that arise from a defensive and self-protective reaction, perhaps sparked by fear or a perceived threat. When our perceptions are distorted, our moods are often forfeited to the shadowy corners of our minds. For this reason, we should monitor our thoughts and attitudes and dispose of unhealthy clutter. Just as our living quarters require regular cleaning, so does our inner being to rid ourselves of the cobwebs of wayward emotions and the dust of cognitive distortions that clutter our lives, limiting our perspective.

While psychological problems may arise from various causes, they can only persist or worsen when the mind is caught in its own self-generated vortex, mesmerized by irrational beliefs. These beliefs are erroneous judgments or old mental habits, says Alimaras, that usually develop from cognitive distortions. He cites Albert Ellis's position that there are twelve irrational beliefs from which many psychological disorders result. Each belief is identified, and then its rational opposite, which should be substituted in its place. For instance, the notion that psychological difficulties are caused by external events is an erroneous belief that should be replaced by the thought that such problems are, in fact, the result of interpretations we make of events.

This self-help strategy relies in effect on replacing the old, irrational "tape" with a message that makes more sense. It is a form of autosuggestion designed to retrain the cognitive patterns to a more realistic turn. Alimaras observes, "If our thinking is based on irrational patterns, then our feelings will follow suit." Thus emotional disorders are not unlike audiotapes continually playing the same groundless messages over and over. Yet the sanest of persons often replays old tapes—tapes that should have been erased long ago. More often than not, we blame our surroundings and outer circumstances, especially other people, for the way we feel; it's a convenient excuse we habitually retreat behind, a reflex that might be considered a distortion.

In *Attitude and Your Life!* Robert C. Smith states, "If external conditions determined our state of mind, we would all react to similar circumstances in the same way; but we don't." Our individual sensibilities, of course, filter how we react to circumstances, but Smith makes the meaningful observation that we have a great deal more control of our state of mind than we ordinarily realize. This is an important fact to remember while exploring the issue of sleep disorders. An axiom that often appears in the readings, as in 5023-2, is that "no urge in the astrological, in the vocational, in the hereditary or the environmental . . . surpasses the will or determination of the entity." There is one facet of our beings, however, that the will cannot control which even Cayce acknowledged and this is our need to sleep. We can neither will ourselves to sleep nor to remain awake indefinitely.

Whether our perceptions are correct or not, the feelings they cause don't know the difference. And no person can go through life untouched by emotional upsets. Who can claim never to have felt the clutch, however briefly, of anxiety? Who has avoided the cloud of depression? Most of our disturbances, meanwhile, issue from imbalances that occur among body, mind, and spirit, as the readings suggest. Alimaras studied Cayce's psychic commentaries in light of his training as a psychologist and wrote:

> The psychological problem then is multifaceted and has spiritual, mental, and physical determinants. Spiritual factors interface with the body's en-

docrine system, while mental factors interface with the autonomic nervous system. As spirit, mind, and body are interdependent and interact with each other, the treatment approach of the readings is holistic. It addresses a system in conflict and assumes that little can be accomplished otherwise. Attempts to work with habits at the level of immediate causation may prove fruitless, as they always relate to more remote factors within the system. Although symptom relief can occur by dealing with immediate causes, the cure may be temporary. This was evident in certain readings where the sleeping Cayce asked why the individuals were seeking help. If they wanted freedom from suffering and a return to their normal lifestyles, the readings indicated that it was these very styles that produced their problems in the first place. This idea can be likened to someone who is on a crash diet, only to return to the former eating patterns once the goal is accomplished and regain the weight.

Edgar Cayce, of course, could assume the exceptional psychic insight to fathom the cause behind any disturbance. He could also read people's commitment not only to become well but also their determination to remain healthy. This contradiction prevails with many people. On the one hand we want to be healed and on the other we want to continue our old habits and lifestyles, which impaired our health in the first place. The same opposing inclinations ultimately will foil a person's efforts to find a cure for insomnia.

Two of the most prevalent emotional difficulties that are banes to sleep are anxiety and depression. The extent of these conditions ranges from small doses to landslides; and there is no one who is exempt from feeling their presence.

Anxiety

If there is one thing capable of playing havoc with your emotions and can cause you to toss and turn all night, it is anxiety. It might be said that anxiety is worry run amok. To a psychologist, anxiety is a special form of fear, an intense feeling of mental dread. Anxiety generally is taken to mean that the anticipated threat or danger is not clearly known. The person in the throes of anxiety expects to be overwhelmed by some future event. Chronic anxiety is considered a mental disorder when it is groundless, with no connection to reality, and disrupts the person from functioning normally. It is a symptom of a number of mental disturbances, including schizophrenia and obsessive-compulsive neuroses. When it comes to anxiety disorders, the feeling of anxiety is sometimes the only symptom. Physical, psychological, and behavioral symptoms accompany panic attacks. The physical reactions are powerful and many, including pounding heart, sweating palms, rapid breathing, dizziness, headaches, diarrhea, cramps, sexual dysfunction, and of course insomnia.

A number of disturbances come under the heading of anxiety disorders, but the cause of the condition is not clear. The spectrum of theories ranges from the explanation that the disorder is a learned one or that it arises from physical causes. From the vantage of the Cayce psychic information, fear is both the source of more trouble than any other influence in a person's experience and the root cause of most of our human ills. His advice to those beset by personal problems was to avoid worry and anxiousness. In reading 1472-7, he likened anxiety to fear, "and is as canker to any disturbed *nervous* condition of a body, if it takes hold."

Cayce found various causes for anxiety, including physical injuries and experiences in previous lifetimes. In a reading for a forty-four-year-old man (3318-1) who wanted to know whether his anxiety was caused by early childhood fears, as psychoanalysts believed. Cayce assured him that this was not the case, that the problem ensued from his having been struck on the right side by a baseball bat, which had injured his cerebrospinal nerves. A fifty-four-year-old woman (823-1) was told that her early childhood phobic reaction to spiders and knives was connected to the subconscious memory of experiences in a previous lifetime in France.

While recommendations were offered to individuals according to the specifics of their cases, there was one suggestion given frequently when others were facing situations that put them in a fretful frame of mind. The sleeping Cayce would ask, "Why worry when you can pray?" And in reading 3569-1, he specifically warned, "When you can't pray—you'd better begin to worry! For then you have something to worry about!" It goes without saying that prayer has the power to effect physical consequences as well as spiritual, as those who rely on it during difficult periods have come to discover. Alimaras considers prayer a powerful element that can bring positive improvements and combine effectively with psychological strategies.

"Fear springs from a misunderstanding of the soul's relationship with God . . . " writes Smith, citing the Cayce readings. As a result—and in the process—we identify exclusively with the temporal world, giving our trust to things transitory; in effect, "We lose sight of our identity as God's children . . . " Prayer, then, is an acknowledgment of our relationship to the Creator. Prayer and meditation together form a two-way connection. By the former, we speak with God; and through the silence of the latter, God speaks to us. In this way it is possible to receive divine help and healing.

Depression

If fear is a failure of spirit, then depression is a dark night of the soul. If you have ever gone through a spell of true depression—even a minor episode—you know a feeling of dejection or sadness is only one of several symptoms. In some cases, the person may not be aware in the least of feeling sad. Clinical depression includes loss of incentive, poor concentration, diminished energy, feelings of hopelessness, and self-destructive thoughts, as well as other symptoms. Sleep is disturbed, of course, typically by awakening too early. While other symptoms occur, not every individual experiences all of them. Some develop increased appetite, and others entirely lose the desire for food.

Like anxiety, depression affects your mind, body, and behavior. Occasionally, it is found to be a symptom of some other disorder. In some cases, it is accompanied by anxiety, and when depression seesaws with hyperactive moods, it is defined as bipolar or manic-depression disorder. Periods of normal sadness may be caused by the death of someone close, but in most cases they do not pose a major problem to the individual. Out of a population of a million people, 1,400 men suffer from depression; the number of women skyrockets to 4,000. The disorder increases in men as they age, but studies reveal that most depressed women will experience it during their mid-thirties to mid-forties. Experts speculate that the higher number of reported cases among women may indicate that they are more inclined to seek help than men.

Numerous queries regarding depression came to Cayce from people apparently suffering from this mood disorder. From the psychic perspective, attention in many cases was primarily directed to low self-esteem and the sense of worthlessness exhibited by these individuals.

The lexicon of the readings defines self-condemnation as an expression of selfishness. Smith remarks that condemnation involves "the imposition of judicial sentence or some other penalty." Recognition and admission of wrongdoing can end guilt, but "Condemnation goes beyond this and demands punishment. This is what makes depression terribly destructive. Self-condemnation is self-judgment that can lead to self-destruction."

A young woman (2540-1), who worked as a showgirl and model, asked Cayce why she was always thinking about killing herself. The reply included the reminder that she had not given enough attention to expressing God's will. Cayce made it clear that just as we have no right to judge others neither do we have the right to judge ourselves. The besetting sin of humankind, according to the readings, is *self* and includes those characteristics that express themselves through the ego—selfishness, self-aggrandizement, self-glorification, etc., which are exulted in at the expense of others. Self-preoccupation breeds conflict between the soul's impulses and the ego's urges. This state of affairs, in turn, brings about imbalances recorded in body, mind, and spirit and that eventually reveal themselves as mental and emotional disorders. Cayce looked upon body, mind, and soul as one. So whatever affects any one of these has an impact on the other two facets of our beings. To abuse one is to abuse all.

Despite the fact that depression, as with anxiety, is a mood disorder, it can originate in any of the three facets of our beings. And just as he found with anxiety, Cayce also traced some depression cases to physical problems, spinal injuries in particular. One woman (964-1) was advised that her depression was induced by the aftereffects of giving birth. Another [1133] was told that her disturbance—periods of melancholia as well as the inability to sleep—arose from conditions produced by menopause.

The spiritual element, from the standpoint of the readings, is always an integral part of an illness and its treatment. With mental and emotional disorders in particular, the spiritual becomes paramount in facing a difficulty and overcoming it, an experience which takes us back to the idea that constructive attitudes and emotions become stepping stones to health and balance. And also to a good night's sleep.

Constructive Change

If you are prone to depression, anxiety, or any undesirable attitude or behavioral problem, help clearly is as close as your own thoughts and attitudes. Remember Cayce's assurance that no urge surpasses your will or determination. Smith offers the reminder that our mental and spiritual well-being are not based solely on eliminating negatives such as fear and guilt. The negatives must be supplanted with positives. To that end, he provides prayers, affirmations, and visualizations to counter each undesirable attitude discussed in his book. These are the catalysts for constructive change.

Most of us still don't get the idea of free will. Within the realm of our individual beings, nothing supersedes it. True, circumstances sometimes appear beyond our control, but they do not control us. The following story is a case in point. It is a wonderful testament to the will—and the human heart—committed to the highest expression of love. George G. Ritchie, Jr., M.D., was a medic in World War II. In 1943, he underwent a near-death experience during which he was in the presence of the Christ. From this experience, he made it a practice to try to see the spirit of Christ in everyone he met. That spirit was never more evident than in a man Ritchie met at the end of the war. The following is taken from his book, *Return from Tomorrow*:

When the war in Europe ended in May 1945, the 123rd Evac entered Germany with the occupying troops. I was part of a group assigned to a concentration camp near Wuppertal, charged with getting medical help to the newly liberated prisoners, many of them Jews from Holland, France, and eastern Europe. This was the most shattering experience I had yet had; I had been exposed many times by then to sudden death and injury, but to see the effects of slow starvation, to walk through those barracks where thousands of men had died a little bit at a time over a period of years, was a new kind of horror. For many it was an irreversible process: we lost scores each day in spite of all the medicine and food we could rush to them.

Now I needed my new insight indeed. When the ugliness became too great to handle, I did what I had learned to do. I went from one end to the other of that barbed wire enclosure looking into men's faces until I saw looking back at me the face of the Christ.

And that's how I came to know Wild Bill Cody. That wasn't his real name. His real name was seven unpronounceable syllables in Polish, but he had long drooping handlebar mustaches like a picture of the old western hero, so the American soldiers called him Wild Bill. He was one of the inmates of the concentration camp, but obviously he hadn't been there long: his posture was erect, his eyes bright, his energy indefatigable. Since he was fluent in English, French, German, and Russian, as well as Polish, he became a kind of unofficial camp translator.

We came to him with all sorts of problems; the paper work alone was staggering in attempting to relocate people whose families, even whole hometowns, might have disappeared. But though Wild Bill worked fifteen and sixteen hours a day, he showed no signs of weariness. While the rest of us were drooping with fatigue, he seemed to gain strength. "We have time for this old fellow," he'd say. "He's been waiting to see us all day." His compassion for his fellow-prisoners glowed on his face, and it was to this glow that I came when my own spirits were low.

So I was astonished to learn when Wild Bill's own papers came before us one day that he had been in Wuppertal since 1939! For six years he had lived on the same starvation diet, slept in the same airless and disease-ridden barracks as everyone else, but without the least physical or mental deterioration.

Perhaps even more amazing, every group in the camp looked on him as a friend. He was the one to whom quarrels between inmates were brought for arbitration. Only after I'd been at Wuppertal a number of weeks did I realize what a rarity this was in a compound where the different nationalities of prisoners hated each other almost as much as they did the Germans.

As for the Germans, feeling against them ran so high that in some of the camps liberated earlier, former prisoners had seized guns, run into the nearest village, and simply shot the first Germans they saw. Part of our instructions were to prevent this kind of thing and again Wild Bill was our greatest asset, reasoning with the different groups, counseling forgiveness.

"It's not easy for some of them to forgive," I commented to him one day as we sat over mugs of tea in the processing center. "So many of them have lost members of their families."

Wild Bill leaned back in the upright chair and sipped at his drink. "We lived in the Jewish section of Warsaw," he began slowly, the first words I had heard him speak about himself, "my wife, our two daughters, and our three little boys. When the Germans reached our street, they lined everyone against a wall and opened up with machine guns. I begged to be allowed to die with my family, but because I spoke German they put me in a work group."

He paused, perhaps seeing again his wife and five children. "I had to decide right then," he continued, "whether to let myself hate the soldiers who had done this. It was an easy decision, really. I was a lawyer. In my practice I had seen too often what hate could do to people's minds and bodies. Hate had just killed the six people who mattered most to me in the world. I decided then that I would spend the rest of my life—whether it was a few days or many years—loving every person I came in contact with."

Loving every person . . . this was the power that had kept a man well in the face of every privation. It was the Power I had first met in a hospital room in Texas, and was learning little by little to recognize wherever He chose to shine through—whether the human vehicle was aware of Him or not.

This account speaks for itself, but the ramifications reach to the heart of the human condition. While it dramatizes that the meanest and most tragic circumstances may intrude, how you face them makes all the difference in the world. Wild Bill's choice, above all, demonstrates that we all have access to that same spirit—regardless of what we call it, and our religious beliefs notwithstanding.

Taking a personal inventory, identifying destructive attitudes and emotions, and changing them comprise the first step in adopting a disposition conducive to sleep, and especially to quality sleep. A kind of magic occurs when you assume a more positive outlook and stop generating negative feelings: Things begin to change, your life is less frustrating, and often your very circumstances are transformed. Also, the pace and rhythm of your life ease back on the throttle to a more tolerable tempo. Constructive change requires an attitude of cooperation, a decision to think and act in accord with your highest purpose, and a commitment to live your physical, mental, and spiritual ideals. The pace and rhythm of your life turn on the axle of these personal dynamics. And those same dynamics have a direct bearing on how well you sleep. To that end, if there is one rhythm we should cooperate with to advantage, it's our circadian rhythm.

Circadian Rhythms

All of nature, all life, is allied with cycles keyed by inner responses to the natural world. The human body has more than 100 cycles or rhythms, such as breathing, heartbeat, temperature, and sleep. These physical cycles are cued to the solar day of twenty-four hours and are referred to as circadian rhythms. Cayce observed that every cell of the body is like a tiny universe. And scientists now believe that each cell possesses its own clock, and apparently different parts of cells have clocks capable of functioning separately, if necessary. Researchers have found that a section of tissue from a living organism will adhere to its own clock rhythm and then will readjust to the organism's clock when rejoined with it. This has been demonstrated experimentally by removing and replacing the eye of a sea slug.

In 1998, researchers at the University of North Carolina at Chapel Hill discovered a new light-sensitive pigment in the brain, eye, and skin. The pigment apparently regulates the circadian rhythm in mammals. Until this finding, according to researcher Dr. Aziz Sancar, "[I]t was assumed that the same pigment was responsible for both vision and circadian synchronization. We have now shown that is not true." The pigments, called cryptochromes, come in two forms and are located in separate parts of the retina. Thus, a blind person who loses part of the retina while retaining the section with the circadian pigment can remain synchronized to a normal rhythm.

The biochemical processes carried on in the body are highly complex, and science has a great deal yet to learn. The information gleaned from the study of our biological clocks will be of immeasurable benefit to science. Among other areas of interest, the workings of our clocks will help researchers understand how these internal timers affect aging. All animals appear to have a master clock in their brains that communicates chemically with other parts of the body. The hormone melatonin, which is found in the pineal gland where it is produced in reaction to darkness, is believed to play a major part in regulating the body's circadian rhythm. The biological clocks enable us—and other creatures—to function in harmony with the cycles of nature. The plant kingdom obviously follows circadian rhythms. There are other types of cycles, such as infradian rhythms, which are monthly rather than daily timers found in the ovulation of female mammals. A woman's clock, for example, is timed according to a succession of hormonal secretions—from the ovary, hypothalamus, and pituitary—which determines the monthly cycle. Seasonal changes occur in nature, of course, as in people who suffer from seasonal affective disorder (SAD), a period of extreme depression resulting from insufficient exposure to bright light in the fall and winter. Daily exposure to bright or full-spectrum lighting usually corrects the illness.

Light is the key synchronization element in adapting our rhythms to the twenty-four-hour cycle. Our bodies are cued for sleep during one-third of the day—the darkest hours under normal circumstances. It is easy to foul up the synchronization of the sleep-wake cycle. Many people do it inadvertently. You have to keep in mind that our world today is much brighter in the evenings than it was 100 years ago. This is why, if you have difficulty getting to sleep at night, you should avoid bright or direct lighting for a couple of hours before bedtime. It is also a good idea to turn off the television an hour or so before bedtime. Some sleep therapists discourage reading prior to turning in; but if you do read, it should be material that does not overstimulate your mind or emotions.

Obviously, maintaining your rhythm is the key to preventing lost sleep. But circumstances can force you to reset your clock to a different pattern from your normal schedule. Jet lag and night work are two of the most common intrusions that force the hands of the internal clock out of synchronization. Many people find common-sense solutions to these changes without having to consult a sleep therapist. Anyone whose body is healthy will usually be able to adapt without much difficulty.

For jet lag, there is a simple way to adjust your internal clock to the new time zone. When you arrive at your destination, soak in a tub of warm water (not hot) for fifteen minutes. Then, lie down and rest or nap for twenty to thirty minutes. If you arrive early in the day, you can extend your nap to an hour. In the evening go to bed at about your usual time. If you arrive late in the day, a quick soak and a nap will pep you up; you should be able to adjust by the following day to your new time. People who have to work nights realize two things are paramount: quiet and dark surroundings. Yet even under the most suitable conditions, staying up all night and then sleeping during the day is putting the cart before the horse to say the least, and it is difficult to get the quality of sleep provided by a normal circadian rhythm. One thing night workers should be aware of is they are at risk of suffering from SAD, and should make sure they get adequate exposure to light. If necessary, they should follow a regimen of light therapy treatments.

Aging and Sleep

Your sleep pattern changes as you age. A common complaint among the elderly is waking up in the middle of the night after only a few hours. People in their seventies often experience several awakenings. One of the reasons may be that the pineal's production of melatonin, which is in abundant supply when we are young, dwindles with age. Older people are light sleepers because they spend less time in the deep stages of sleep. The National Institute on Aging recommends that if you experience a change in your sleep pattern to consult your doctor. The following suggestions are adapted from the Institute's "Age Page" and provides helpful tips to anyone wanting a good night's sleep—good advice regardless of your age:

- Go to bed and get up at the same time each day.
- Moderate exercise at least two hours before turning in will aid sleep.
- Get some exposure to natural light in the afternoon.
- Avoid coffee, tea, or colas late in the day.
- Don't smoke or drink alcohol to help you sleep. Alcohol can disrupt sleep, and nicotine is a stimulant. Do not smoke in bed or when you feel sleepy.
- Make your home as safe and as comfortable as possible—with locks on all doors and smoke alarms on every floor. An easy-to-reach bedside lamp and a dark, quiet, and well-ventilated room with a phone next to your bed will help you feel secure and aid relaxation.
- Follow a regular routine prior to bedtime each night, such as reading or soaking in a tub.
- Use your bed for sleep only. If you are not asleep in

fifteen minutes after turning off the light and don't feel drowsy, then get up and go to another room until you do feel drowsy.

- Do not worry about sleep. Dwell on pleasant thoughts or play mental games. Convince yourself that you have to get up in five minutes and just need a few extra winks.

The Institute includes this advisory: "If you are so tired during the day that you cannot function normally and this fatigue lasts for more than two or three weeks, you should see your family doctor or a sleep disorders specialist for a complete evaluation."

As people grow older, they become prime candidates for insomnia because they often fail to get enough restorative sleep. They remain in the upper stages of sleep without settling for long into stages three and four or shifting into REM sleep, which is necessary for a revitalizing rest. And for the elderly, getting a restful night's sleep is often complicated by physical ailments and by the sleep-robbing aches and pains that come with them. The situation is compounded when the illness requires medications, especially those containing caffeine or other stimulants. There are also numerous drugs that cause insomnia. At the same, older people are prone to use sleeping pills more often than younger adults. More on these subjects next.

BEHIND THE MIRROR

A funny thing happened on the way to this modern age. It is still happening: We are seemingly beset by an ever-increasing number of diseases and ailments, or maybe we just got better at isolating and identifying the sources of our complaints.

The good news is that we have developed numerous medicines and drugs as our chemical forts to ward off unseen viral and other undesirable barbarians at the gates of our health. And these concoctions of medical science have triumphed over many of the invaders. By the time Jonas Salk developed his famous polio vaccine against that crippling disease, we already knew where to find relief for countless other serious and milder complaints. Behind every medicine cabinet mirror in the world the shelves became stocked with magic formulas in bottles.

These formulas are comprised of not only prescription drugs but a plethora of over-the-counter medicines as well. Some of these chemicals, of course, are vital maintenance prescriptions related to serious ailments such as heart disease, asthma, diabetes. But most are nonprescription medicines kept on hand as ready reserves against future internal skirmishes—aspirin, antacids, cough syrups, decongestants, and sleeping pills, to name a few.

This brings us to the bad news. The 1900s also saw an increasing tendency for people to rely on a quick fix to alleviate uncomfortable symptoms, as if quelling discomfort is enough. Instead of seeing a headache, for example, as a sign that attention should be given to some aspect of their bodies or habits, millions of people settle for relieving the symptoms with an over-the-counter potion without regard to the causes. To coin a name for it, let's call this habit the Stop the Symptom Syndrome (SSS): the mistaken idea that treating symptoms is enough to dispel the problem. In the case of harmless ailments, temporary relief buys time for the cause to settle down. But in other cases suppressing symptoms may be hazardous to your health—not to mention your life. While most people know this, too many insist on pushing the envelope of risk. This is the reason people sometimes die because they gobble down antacids for heartburn, when, in fact, they are having a heart attack, and the delay or failure to get treatment ends tragically.

During a siege of illness, of course, symptoms loom large. After all, it's the symptoms that get your attention, particularly those that produce acute pain or discomfort; the cause itself is often hidden or difficult to trace. When you are aching with pain, obviously the first order of business is relief. Yet once relief is provided, you are inclined to put the problem behind you. Meanwhile, there is nothing new about SSS. It is a modern expression of our resistance to changing our habits. This resistance bears on a question Edgar Cayce sometimes asked—in effect: Do you want to get well so that you can go back and do the things that made you sick in the first place?

Sleep from a Bottle

When you can't sleep, downing a pill or two seems to be the simplest and surest remedy. Insomnia has become such a prevalent complaint worldwide that more and more people are driven by frustration and desperation to find relief in a pill. Never mind the drug's contents and the possible reactions. The insomniac wants sleep at any price. But it should be kept in mind that insomnia is a symptom.

There are also a number of problems that come with the use of sleeping pills. Most of these drugs quickly lose effectiveness if taken for more than a couple of weeks. Extended use can also result in addiction, because the body develops a tolerance, and thus requires a larger dosage to have any effect. Then there are the side effects sleeping pills produce that carry over during the day— fatigue, fuzzy thinking, poor coordination. Peter Hauri reports in *No More Sleepless Nights* that dozens of studies confirm that "When performance tasks such as driving simulations were assessed after nights on pills and nights on placebo, the pills often impaired performances the next day even more than a night of poor sleep."

Sleeping pills are dangerous for a number of reasons. Consuming them over long periods can bring on serious side effects, among them liver and kidney ailments, high blood pressure, loss of appetite, digestive problems, depression, anxiety, and damage to the central nervous system. To add insult to injury, sleeping pills do not help you get a good night's sleep. For one thing, studies show that these drugs suppress REM sleep. For another, they prevent the sleeper from reaching stage four at all. These two stages are required for the body to get any semblance of true restoration during the hours of unconsciousness. It was also found that subjects who used the pills awoke more often during the night than those who did not take them. These are some of the many reasons people are always cautioned not to take any drugs without first seeking the advice of their physicians.

When stage-four sleep is curtailed or disturbed, you wake up stiff and achy. Sleeping pills are not the only culprits that upset the normal sleep cycle; many drugs interfere with the deepest stage of sleep. Tranquilizers cause you to linger too long in the first stage, thus steal valuable time needed for the fourth stage. According to research findings, however, muscle relaxants apparently do not disturb this stage.

A great many things can affect your sleep, and not all are easily detected. The following Cayce reading reveals a cause for insomnia most of us would never think of; and it also attests to the validity of modern research on the inadvisability of taking drugs for insomnia. A fifty-seven-year-old woman (1711-1) asked Edgar Cayce what she could do to enable her to sleep through the night. Cayce informed her that removing the impurities in her body would "relieve the tensions upon the nervous system in such a way that the functions of the body will bring the normal rest . . . " This reading included specific recommendations for cleaning her intestinal tract, along with directions for taking Atomidine and vitamins following the internal cleansing. He added that this approach was preferable to relying on drugs—unless necessary for pain—because sleep induced by artificial means "is not a *natural* rest, nor does it produce a regeneration for the activities of the physical body."

Physical strain on the woman's nervous system occurred from the body's struggle to fight the effects of and rid itself of drosses. To assist the body in its housecleaning effort, the reading specified a mixture of compounds to flush out the impurities. As with many of Cayce's psychic diagnoses, the wisdom of this reading is that the cause, though hardly obvious, was identified, which eliminated guesswork in offering guidance for appropriate treatment. A more conventional diagnosis, on the other hand, might have addressed only the symptom and prescribed medication that had no real curative value in cleaning the impurities from her system. Perhaps it should be noted, too, that drugs themselves often become impurities in the body, considering that they are rarely substances natural to the body's chemistry, but are foreign agents imposed on it.

Quitting the Pill Habit

Sleeping pills are a perniciously double-edged sword. There are risks in taking them, and there are complications when quitting after becoming dependent on them. It is a peculiar fact that you can remain addicted to them although they do not benefit your sleep whatsoever. If you have suddenly quit a sleep drug you were dependent on, your insomnia likely became worse than it was before you started using the drug. You experienced rebound insomnia, a symptom that went away when you resumed the habit. Quitting suddenly, however, can also produce other symptoms—anxiety, cramps, depression, and nausea.

If you believe you may be addicted to sleeping pills (and you *are* if you cannot quit without experiencing distressing symptoms), you would be wise to talk with your doctor, who will likely recommend and provide treatment for slow withdrawal from your habit. If you are considering taking sleeping pills, see your doctor. If you are thinking of taking any of the numerous over-the-

counter sleep drugs without your doctor's knowledge—
don't. And keep in mind that for short-term use there are
safer alternatives. These will be discussed later.

Not surprisingly, the science of pharmacology is
unimaginably complex, especially when it comes to the
intricate dynamics of drugs and how they affect the body,
not to mention the interactions among different drugs.
The riskiest group of drugs is probably the most commonly prescribed: antibiotics. Penicillin reportedly is responsible for several hundred deaths each year—which
adds new meaning to the idea that the cure is worse than
the illness. It is estimated that lethal reactions are more
likely to result from drugs than poisonous insect bites. In
many instances, allergic drug reactions begin with mild
symptoms, perhaps swelling of the face or an outbreak of
a few hives, then progress to more serious conditions,
including difficulty breathing and even heart tremors.

The pharmacology team of Joe and Teresa Graedon
offers excellent advice to help you protect yourself from
the possibility of harmful drug interactions. In their best-
selling book, *The People's Guide to Deadly Drug Interactions*, they recommend that you:

- Take charge of your own health. In the end, you are
responsible for the pills you take. Inform all your doctors
about all drugs you are taking, and make sure they check
for possible interactions by consulting the reference books
and computer programs containing this information.
- Rely on your pharmacists, who are trained professionals and specialists in the field of drugs and interactions. Provide them with a complete list of all medications
you are taking, and tell them you want to know about
any possible incompatibility.
- Report any unusual symptoms to your doctor immediately. The Graedons suggest never starting or stopping a medication without your doctor's supervision.

"Stopping certain medications suddenly," they explain, "could trigger irregular heart rhythms, not to mention convulsion or heart attacks. In addition, discontinuing one drug may have a domino effect, in that it could increase or decrease the effects of other medicines you may be taking."

- Be aware that the U.S. Food and Drug Administration (FDA) has no organized system for monitoring drug interactions and no effective method of informing doctors. The *Physicians' Desk Reference* contains some dangerous reactions, though not all, while it can take years for this information to be included in standard reference books.

- Do not presume no information is good news. It's possible for lethal interactions to go unrecognized for months and even years. "If you are experiencing a strange or dangerous symptom that cannot easily be explained," the Graedons advise, "ask your physician to contact the drug's manufacturer and to file a report with the FDA.

To the above advice, it might be added that no one under a doctor's care should be resigned to a passive role. It is far wiser to follow Norman Cousins's example. Suffering from a debilitating illness that threatened to cripple him and written off by some specialists, Cousins decided to take an interest in his own case and—in evaluating the effect of the painkilling drugs he was taking— he found a better way to deal with the pain and literally laughed himself back to health. Approximately 7,000 patients die annually because of errors involving drugs, and medical blunders in hospitals kill almost 100,000 persons each year, according to the Institute of Medicine. To avoid being an obituary statistic, we all need to communicate thoroughly and carefully with our doctors. Then at least we can sleep a little better on that account.

Drugs that Affect Sleep

Consider the following common drugs. They are a random sampling chosen from a larger group of medications that, aside from their uses, have one thing in common: They affect your sleep. See if you can guess exactly what is the impact of each on your sleep. The information given below for each medication should not be considered as exhaustive:

- **Codeine**—a narcotic analgesic used to treat pain. Also prescribed as an antitussive to control coughing as well as other conditions. Possible allergic reactions: breathing problems, dizziness, hives, severe rash. Possible side effects: constipation, dizziness, excessive drowsiness, headache, lightheadedness, nausea, vomiting.

- **Darvocet**—an analgesic combination (propoxyphene and acetaminophen) prescribed for pain. Some possible side effects: constipation, dizziness, drowsiness, lightheadedness, nausea, vomiting.

- **Halcion**—a benzodiazepine used for treating sleep disorders and other conditions. Possible side effects: clumsiness, dizziness, excessive daytime drowsiness, headache, lightheadedness, unsteadiness, unusual weakness.

- **Librium**—a benzodiazepine used to treat anxiety, alcohol withdrawal, and other conditions. Possible side effects: clumsiness, dizziness, excessive daytime drowsiness, headache, lightheadedness, unsteadiness, unusual weakness.

- **Percodan**—an analgesic combination (oxycodone and aspirin) to prevent or ease moderate to severe pain. Possible allergic reactions: breathing difficulties, dizziness, hives, severe rash, etc. Possible side effects: constipation, blurred vision, dizziness, excessive drowsiness, heartburn, lightheadedness.

- **Restoril**—a benzodiazepine prescribed for sleep disorders and other conditions. Possible side effects: clumsiness, dizziness, excessive daytime drowsiness, lightheadedness, unsteadiness, unusual daytime weakness.
- **Valium**—a benzodiazepine for the treatment of anxiety, alcohol withdrawal, muscle spasms, and other conditions such as seizures and insomnia. Possible side effects: clumsiness, dizziness, excessive daytime drowsiness, headache, lightheadedness, unusual weakness, unsteadiness.
- **Vicodin**—an analgesic combination (hydrocodone and acetaminophen) for the relief of pain. Possible side effects: constipation, dizziness, drowsiness, lightheadedness, nausea, vomiting.

These medications are prescribed by doctors for the conditions indicated. All of them—including the two used primarily for sleep disorders—disturb stage-four sleep. None of these or similar prescription drugs may be in your medicine cabinet, but there are other over-the-counter drugs that can erode the deepest stage of sleep. More than likely you keep a bottle of aspirin on hand. While a couple of aspirin before bed help you get some shut-eye, especially in getting you through the second half of the night without interruption, they also create an imbalance among the sleep stages—more time in stage two, less in stages three and four. This no doubt is partly what Cayce meant when he suggested that using drugs was not the same as natural sleep.

And when it comes to the treatments recommended by the readings, they are above all natural; this is the guiding principle behind the Cayce medical information. The treatments hold special appeal for people who prefer drugless and noninvasive therapies. This body of clairvoyantly derived material introduced America—albeit a small audience in the beginning—to the body-mind-spirit connection when it comes to health and illness. Implicitly the body is not simply the incidental abode of mind. In fact, the mind is the chief engineer of its physical domain and serves as a vital alliance in the health of the body. Cayce always considered the mental state of the person needing help. Consider the following reading:

In 1941, a woman wrote to Edgar Cayce requesting a reading for her seventy-seven-year-old mother [2538], who had been suffering from arteriosclerosis for about six months. Her doctor considered the elderly woman to be in good physical shape "except for her dementia condition," wrote the daughter. The mother did not sleep well at night and, because she was inclined to wander, had to be given sleeping pills and locked in her room unless someone could watch her. In addition to receiving sedatives, she was given iodide shots by a doctor. The daughter was obviously at her wits' end when she wrote, "Is there any cure for it [arteriosclerosis and senile dementia symptoms]? If so, what? Should we place her in a sanitarium?"

Cayce's subconscious mind found the mother's condition to be very serious. He saw that she could be helped "in the physical *and* the mental reactions—if there can and will be something of a desire aroused in the purpose of this entity . . . " He found that her vital energies were deficient, which he likened to a run-down battery, a reference to "the nerve energy in the centers between the cerebrospinal and the sympathetic nerve system." (2538-1) This state was responsible for her physical weakness and irrational reactions.

The reading deemed the treatments she was receiving as beneficial, though the effects were not consistent, and recommended discontinuing the iodide injections, which were replaced by Atomidine taken orally. Cayce noted an important difference between the two iodine preparations: "This atomic iodine, non-poisonous, will react the same upon *all* the glands of the body . . . " Detailed instructions were provided for taking the Atomidine, which was to be alternated with a gold chloride/soda water solution. These were to be taken in the mornings. In the evenings, before bedtime, [2538] was to receive a peanut oil massage from the base of the skull to the end of her spine, using as much oil as the body would absorb.

Vitamin B-1 supplements were also recommended, to be administered under the direction of a doctor—but, Cayce stressed, "*not* by injection." Foods rich in B-1 and iron were also recommended to provide nerve-building energies and properties. A follow-up reading found some improvement in the woman's condition. Further information was given for continuing the treatment, and additional procedures were suggested. No further readings were given, and according to the records the woman died a few years later.

The guidance given for the woman's treatment steered away from the invasive injections altogether, substituting the iodide shots with Atomidine taken orally. Also note Cayce's punctuating the mental responses and his implication that healing depended on awakening a sense of purpose within the woman. Apparently in her drained and disoriented condition, she was lacking in motivation of any kind and did not have the necessary responsiveness to be interested in anything. The impression this reading gives is that the woman possessed only the faintest connection to her own will to live.

The observation regarding purpose—as touched on in the previous chapter—appears throughout the Cayce readings. It is through intentionality that, as Edgar Cayce said numerous times, mind is the builder. When all is said and done, mind as well as body determines how well you sleep. Body and mind—the seen and the unseen—share a symbiotic relationship in the most intimate sense, and what affects one affects the other. Consider the following answer when a fifty-year-old woman asked whether she should continue taking hydrochloric acid internally. She added that she felt better from using it. From his body-mind perspective Cayce replied, "If that is the desire of the body . . . For the mental outlook has as much to do with the results as the material applications!" (1259-2)

Drugs and Aging

The problem for older people is that they are more prone to getting caught in a damned-if-you-do-and-damned-if-you-don't web with regard to drugs. They are likely to suffer from illnesses that disrupt sleep, thus have no choice but to take drugs that undermine the quality of their sleep. They may suffer from such conditions as Alzheimer's disease, arthritis, cancer, dementia, heart failure, incontinence—all of which prevent a good night's rest. At the same time, it is difficult to fall asleep when you are in pain or have trouble breathing.

It is estimated that half the patients with congestive heart failure experience sleep apnea. This disorder is associated with snoring, and when it occurs, breathing halts, blood oxygen levels drop, and then the sleeper wakes momentarily and gasps for air. Breathing can stop for as long as two minutes. A person with this disorder may not recall waking at all; and it is possible for this cycle to repeat itself hundreds of times during the night, while the patient may recall waking only a few times. Sleep apnea appears occasionally in younger adults, but it is found more often among older people who are also obese; and the condition occurs mostly in adults more than sixty years of age. It is more common in men than in women. An estimated twenty-five percent of adults older than sixty-five suffer from the breathing disorder. People who have suffered a stroke or brain tumor or who have cardiac or vascular disease are especially at risk. Smokers, heavy drinkers, and users of mind-altering drugs are also likely to experience sleep apnea.

Apnea has two causes. One is the result of the upper air passageway closing because of anatomical problems. The other is caused by a communications breakdown when the part of the brain responsible for breathing seemingly goes to sleep and stops signaling. The disorder is treacherous; you can suffer from the condition and not be aware of it, unless someone who sleeps in the same bed or room gives you a clue. If you believe you sleep well and through the night, yet you feel sleepy during the day, you may have apnea. You might want to have someone observe you while you sleep to determine whether your breathing stops for more than ten seconds. This and other sleep-robbing disorders should not go untreated. Anyone who experiences apnea should get help from a sleep therapist.

When it comes to drugs, older people present unique challenges for medical professionals in a number of ways. The possibility of suffering an adverse drug reaction increases as you grow older. Your odds are three times those of a younger person. The incidence of adverse reactions in people older than sixty, according to experts, is forty percent. Frequently the reactions are undetected as drug-related. Symptoms may be attributed to another illness or even confused with those of the condition already under treatment. The adverse reaction may be mistakenly attributed to symptoms of aging. And to add a twist to the generation gap, there can be marked differences between a younger patient's reaction to a particular drug and an older person's reaction. There is also the possibility that symptoms caused by reactions may be taken merely as a sign of a disease, such as Alzheimer's.

Drug Reactions and Interactions

Regardless of a person's age, adverse reactions to drugs are always possible. There are more than 300,000 over-the-counter drugs available to consumers in the U.S. It is a selection that invites the temptation of self-medication. There is also temptation in presuming to diagnose yourself, which can be risky and even fatal. Any symptoms that persist over time or continually reoccur should suggest that medical attention is called for. In any case, because a drug is obtainable without a prescription does not mean it is safe for you to take. This is especially true if you are already on another medication—even if both are nonprescription medicines. Taking two drugs at the same time can potentially result in the following: They can combine in a dangerous reaction; they can heighten or reduce the effects of one another; or they can, if similar, amplify the impact on the body. All these effects obviously should be avoided.

Consider a few examples of the detrimental effects of mixing medications. Antacids can reduce drug absorption, for example, or slow down the effects of blood-thinning drugs. In either case, you are being shortchanged. Allergy and cold medicines can intensify the effects of tranquilizers and painkilling drugs. If you mix an antihistamine and sedative, you should hand your car keys to someone else. The action of blood-thinning drugs is increased when aspirin is consumed with them. Aspirin is not as harmless as we assume.

Drug interactions pose complex challenges for doctors and pharmacists alike in keeping you informed of the volatile combinations possible among certain drugs. But as mentioned earlier you bear responsibility in the long run for the drugs you swallow. Whenever you experience an adverse reaction from a drug, regardless of how mild, and especially if it is unexpected, let your doctor know immediately. If you are presently taking drugs for any reason, you—or, if necessary, someone else—should monitor your reactions. Some of the symptoms that can register as adverse reactions to various types of drugs: confusion, constipation, depression, diarrhea, dizziness, extreme drowsiness, incontinence, irritability, nausea, tremors, vomiting, and weakness.

Just as drugs can interact with drugs, certain foods mixed with drugs present further concerns. They can interact to disadvantage by reducing the effectiveness of the drug or depriving the body of nutrients from the food. The combination of certain foods and drugs can backfire with hazardous side effects, and some of the elements in food can create reactions that produce the opposite effect than the medication is intended for. As in the case of mixing different drugs, some foods can either accelerate or slow the effect of a particular drug. Drugs can suppress appetite and even reduce absorption of nutrients, either by expediting eliminations or by inhibiting the assimilation of particular nutrients.

The usual reaction apparently is that food and beverages work against the efficacy of drugs instead of the drugs interfering with the food. The interaction will vary depending upon a person's age, sex, weight, and nutritional health. Some interactions are beneficial rather than detrimental when food and drug combinations work synergistically. For instance, orange and grapefruit juices enhance the absorption of iron from supplements.

Alcohol, Caffeine, Nicotine

Three of the most popular addictive substances—alcohol, caffeine, and nicotine—have been explored and written about widely by researchers. These are the drugs of choice for many millions of people. Each may have a connection to your sleep, and particularly to the quality of your sleep, depending on how you use them.

It must be emphasized that *no medication* should be swallowed with the help of an alcoholic drink. This warning cannot be repeated too often. Twenty-five hundred deaths a year are attributed to alcohol-drug interactions, and almost 50,000 people end up in hospital emergency rooms from carelessly mixing alcohol and drugs. Sleep experts discourage drinking alcohol in any form as a panacea for sleep woes. In some people, in fact, alcohol can keep them awake, which may be the reason insomnia plagues some people in the first place.

Reportedly, beer, wine, and cognac may be exceptions in that they act as sedatives in the body. Nevertheless, the sleep of heavy drinkers is comparable to that of the elderly. Most of the sleep is at the shallow end of unconsciousness and includes frequent awakenings. Deeper sleep eludes them to the detriment of quality sleep, thus interfering with natural slumber. Once the effects of the alcohol wear off, the person wakes up. If you need help getting to sleep, there are better alternatives, which will be discussed momentarily.

If there was ever a substance in the world that is no friend of sleep, it is nature's own stimulant—caffeine. Coffee is the most prevalent source, but numerous products contain caffeine, including soft drinks, chocolate, cocoa, and tea. Even a cup of decaffeinated coffee or tea may have a few milligrams of caffeine. It is also found in some analgesics taken for mild pain and headache. The effect of caffeine is almost immediate once it is in your body. Before you finish drinking a cup of coffee, for example, the caffeine enters the bloodstream and moves to every organ of your body, stimulating your mental acuity and increasing your heartbeat. It also affects other functions, such as increasing the production of digestive acids in the stomach.

Coffee, in particular, poses a difficulty for those struggling with insomnia. They drink it throughout the day to stay awake; and the later in the day they drink coffee, the more likely it will impinge on their sleep. If the caffeine does not keep you awake, having the stimulant in your system will certainly disturb the quality of your sleep. Often, coffee is part of the vicious cycle that develops from dependency on sleeping pills, because the caffeine is needed to shake off the torpor brought on by the drug. A good habit to establish is not to drink coffee after three in the afternoon and to avoid drinking more than two or three cups daily.

Nicotine has similar effects as coffee—speeding up the heart rate and stimulating brain-wave activity. It is no surprise, then, that heavy smokers often have difficulty sleeping through the night. Experts have found heavy smokers and users of smoking and chewing tobacco are in double jeopardy when it comes to getting a decent night's sleep. They commonly have trouble falling asleep because of the stimulation of nicotine in their bodies; and once asleep, withdrawal symptoms may wake them up. Needless to say, the worst and most self-defeating action you can do just before bedtime is to have a final smoke and a cup of coffee. If you are a heavy user of tobacco, curtailing use in the evenings a couple of hours before calling it a night will help.

From the viewpoint of the Cayce information, drugless therapies are the best course. Most of the recommended treatments in the readings seem to entail natural methods. Drugs were rarely considered as a desirable course of action. Injections were shunned in favor of safer alternatives, as indicated earlier. A needle jabbed into the flesh can hardly be considered the body's chosen method of accepting any substance, and Cayce followed an approach agreeable to the body's natural functions. The following offers additional insights into Cayce's clairvoyant view of injections.

A thirty-four-year-old man received a reading from Cayce, who found that incoordination between the sympathetic and cerebrospinal systems produced a series of physical disorders in the man, including dizziness and an irregular heartbeat at times. There were also occasions when the man was blurry-eyed, had difficulties with hearing and speech, and suffered from insomnia. Cayce prescribed a lengthy treatment that involved special fume baths, massage, and dietary suggestions.

During the question-and-answer part of the session, the man wanted to know whether it was possible to regain the hearing in his right ear. Cayce assured him that all his senses would improve with the treatment regimen. Then the man asked, "Were hayfever shots in any way responsible for this trouble?" The psychic replied, "Any shots are responsible for most anything? Yes—they are a part of the disorders." (3629-1)

When questions regarding alcohol, coffee, and tobacco were put to Cayce, the replies were based on a reasonable consideration as to the use of these products. Cayce's advantage over conventional medicine was that he could foresee how an individual would be affected by these, and in all cases he stressed moderation.

Alcohol, as considered in the readings, can be used beneficially and medicinally. It was explained to Miss [275] that within our physical systems fermentation occurs as part of the digestive process. Thus, a small amount of light wine would aid her digestion. In other readings, wine was recommended to be taken with only black or brown bread, but not with meat. Moderation means a few ounces of wine once a day. Well-fermented wines were recommended—meaning neither too sour nor too sweet—such as Tokay, Port, and Sauterne.

And while conceding that whiskey has its place, the readings told Mr. [1467] that it was a poison to his body. Another man, who was receiving electrotherapy treatments at the time, was advised to abstain from all alcoholic drinks, including beer. To make certain the man understood the risks, Cayce explained, "Electricity and alcohol don't work together! It burns tissue, and is not good for *anybody!*" 323-1

Coffee was generally acceptable, according to the psychic commentaries, and if taken without cream or milk, is a food. A moderate amount of sugar with the coffee is fine, but milk with coffee produces a strain on digestion. Under certain circumstances, particularly when a condition exists that bears on eliminations, caffeinated drinks should be avoided. Caffeine, Cayce said, is not digested and in some cases remains in the colon, producing poisons that end up in the system. For some people, combining coffee and meat at the same meal may not be a good idea. When a woman asked Cayce whether coffee was harmful to her body, he replied: "With meats, yes. Without meats, no." (4436-2)

The subject of smoking is also discussed in a number of readings. As with the use of alcohol and caffeine, the password is moderation. Mr. [3539], a middle-aged man, wanted to know which was best for him to smoke: a pipe or cigarettes. The answer: "Smoking in moderation for this body would be helpful. To excess it's very harmful. The smoking of cigarettes is better than most types."

Cayce, of course, was referring to pure tobacco that contains no additives or insecticide residues. He suggested to [303], a fifty-four-year-old woman, that smoking cigarettes would benefit her because they would provide substances "that would counterbalance some of the disturbances in the system. Three to five a day would be correct. This does not necessarily mean that these would be inhaled, but the brand that is of the purer tobacco is the better." (303-23)

Sleep Aids

Let's return to the issue of relying on drugs to induce sleep. It was determined that they are of little benefit. But there are safer alternatives that engender a more natural slumber.

Melatonin, the hormone mentioned earlier, has come to be widely recognized as an effective sleep inducer. Produced by the pineal gland in darkness, it is abundant when you are young, but production wanes with age. The hormone is available as a supplement, which some travelers use to overcome the effects of jet lag and to adjust their sleep cycles to a new time zone. Melatonin is available without prescription in one- and three-milligram tablets. It may be wise to limit its use to only a few nights at most. All the research is not in on this hormone, and its long-term effect is unknown.

A better choice might be valerian, an herb that has been used since ancient times. While it is used these days as a sedative and sleep aid, in the past it was also used for flatulence. Although valerian has been used for many years in other parts of the world, it became widely available in the U.S. only in the last decade. It is sold primarily as a supplement in capsules. This herb can also be prepared as a tea.

According to clinical studies, the herb kava is nonaddictive and safe as an anti-anxiety medication, as well as a pain reliever. It also helps promote restful sleep. Kava is a mild narcotic that improves mood and produces relaxation without harmful side effects. It also aids concentration, memory, and response time for people who suffer from anxiety. As an anti-inflammatory agent, kava is used for treating urinary tract problems and is applied externally in liniment form as an anesthetic and pain reliever.

Another herb, shizandra, helps regulate the central nervous system. A study conducted in China in the 1980s indicated that this herb relieves dizziness, calms a racing heart, and relieves headaches and insomnia. It has also been shown that shizandra makes people more alert and increases physiological responses.

Numerous herbs have been used for the purpose of inducing sleep—almonds, catnip, chamomile, fennel, passion flower, skullcap, and others. What may work for one person, of course, might not work for another. As with all substances, whether natural or synthetic, side effects and allergic reactions are possible. When using any supplement or herb for the first time, it is wise to begin with the smallest dosage to test your own sensitivity and gauge how it affects you.

An age-old homespun remedy for insomnia is warm milk. There is a scientific explanation for why this approach is helpful, at least for some people. The short answer is that calcium is the magician. But warm milk is not a panacea; it is only a palliative to help you relax and take the edge off when you are keyed up. Most people have heard of this elixir for treating sleeplessness, and it has received mixed reviews. Cayce also recommended warm milk, but with what may be called a catalytic addition, as in this advice given to a young woman (2514-7) who wondered why she had trouble sleeping: "This is from nervousness and overanxiety. Of course, keep away from any drugs if possible—though a sedative at times may be necessary. Drink a glass of warm milk with a teaspoonful of honey stirred in same." Try this mixture and you may be surprised at the results. Honey, however, should not be given to infants. A small percentage of honey has been found to contain a type of spore that can cause severe illness in babies. It is not harmful for older children and adults.

If one principle comes through clearly in the readings, it's that enduring health is maintained by a balance of activities and moderation of habits. And health is a con-

tract between the Divine and the physical. It is by attending to these agreements that we maintain our health.
Whenever illness or dis-ease beset us, it is because we
disregard the contract. We know this at the deepest level
of our beings, because if we have persisted in ignoring
balance and moderation, we are reminded every time we
look in the medicine cabinet mirror.

4

FOOD FOR SLEEP—AND THOUGHT

"**Y**ou are what you eat" is an adage that seems to be missing one element, judging by the Cayce readings, which state that the combination of what we think and what we eat makes us what we are. So it is that what we allow ourselves to chew on mentally is as important as the organic substances we devour.

It is a kind of paradox that many people give a great deal of attention and care to the foods they put into their mouths, yet they will allow any stray, riffraff thought into their minds. It may be that most of us, however, are careless on both counts. We eat and think whatever we choose, thus forfeiting moderation and balance to whim, with no thought of the consequences.

Of the two, food and thought, the latter is arguably the most important if we consider the experience of Wild Bill, recounted in chapter 2. We were advised two thousand years ago, in fact, that what comes out of our mouths does us more harm than what goes into it. You will recall the Polish lawyer spent six years in a concentration camp surviving on a starvation diet, yet showed no signs of nutritional deficiency, unlike the other prisoners. Bill, of course, had no choice about what he ate; he apparently accepted his meager portions of food without malice toward his captors. His thinking was dedicated to loving others, everyone without qualification. This made all the difference in the world—and in heaven. By helping others and unequivocally nurturing fellow prisoners, he, in turn, was nurtured with manna from heaven. His experience demonstrates the truth that Spirit answers to spirit. Is there any other explanation?

Physician and author Andrew Weil (*Spontaneous Healing*) observes, "I have seen too many people who have lived to ripe old ages on 'bad' diets to believe that food is the sole or even chief determinant of good health. It is simply one influence, one that we can do something about." Indeed, mundane food alone may not tell the whole story of our existence, but it is the resource the vast majority of us rely on for physical sustenance. Nutrients are the fuels that power the body and maintain its health and vitality. A proper diet contributes to physical balance and well-being, which are the ingredients necessary for the quality sleep you deserve. On the other hand, foods of little or no nutritional value consumed in place of a wholesome diet can eventually wreck your health and slumber.

It is a peculiar dichotomy that you can be well fed and yet suffer from malnutrition. Scientists have probed many of the chemical processes related to the way nutrients are used by the body. We know which foods offer the most nourishment and benefit for the multiplicity of organic functions. During the last several decades while researchers were compiling enough data to fill a small library that documented the most healthful foods to consume, there was also a growing mountain of heat-and-serve foods available, not to mention the proliferation of fast-food eateries that spread virtually around the globe. Despite the nutritional knowledge dished out to us, we have indulged more and more in less than genuinely nourishing food.

We are also in the habit of grabbing nutrient-poor meals cooked in a hurry and gobbling them down on the run. It is a habit that propagates a future nutritional debt, and the payback is bad health. Even when so-called fresh foods are prepared at home, there is no guarantee they are as nutritionally rich as they should be. Many of the fruits and vegetables purchased at the grocery store are harvested before completely ripening or maturing. Thus they are often deprived of a full measure of nutrients—and so are consumers. There is a world of difference, for example, between the quality, and even taste, of a vine-ripened tomato and one picked green and left to ripen off the vine.

Our eating and personal habits have been backfiring for decades. Gastrointestinal disorders are at plague levels and continue spreading like wildfire around the world. One major prescription medication for gastric problems, including heartburn and ulcers, sells each year to the tune of $1.7 billion in the U.S. alone and $3.7 billion worldwide. Antacids and other medicines for stomach ailments are reportedly used by 90 million Americans. Global sales annually for ulcer medications have risen to $8.6 billion, and drugs sales for gastroesophageal reflux disease are at $930 million, while antacids pull in $1.3 billion.

Alarming statistics—enough to give you indigestion. They seem to suggest, among other things, that we are eating all the wrong foods in all the wrong places. Taking into account various other factors that lead us into the valley of the shadow of sickness, anyone might feel this notion sounds a bit simplistic. The health of the body, however, depends upon proper nourishment to fortify it against the threat of disease and stress. Health in body, mind, and spirit equals happiness—and restful sleep. It's very difficult for your mind to stay up to par if your body is undernourished (unless perhaps you're like Wild Bill); and it's impossible for your spirit to enliven the mind if your thoughts are burdened by physical disturbances.

A separate body of literature has practically been built around the importance of food to body-mind functions and interactions. Researchers have found that certain foods are more likely to help our mood than others. Foods rich in tryptophan, one of the essential amino acids, are particularly helpful. Poultry and fish, as well as other meats, have this amino acid in abundance. It is also present in eggs, cheese, milk, sour cream, nuts, soybeans, and leafy vegetables. The body uses tryptophan to produce serotonin, which operates as a neurotransmitter that modulates nerve activity and helps induce sleep. Tryptophan was once available as an over-the-counter supplement, which held promise as a treatment for depression and anxiety. But the U.S. Food and Drug Administration banned sales of the supplement in the late 1980s after a batch became contaminated, causing a rare muscle disorder that affected thousands of users and resulted in the deaths of almost two dozen people. Tryptophan is available now only by prescription and from a pharmacy that specializes in compounding. As a sleep inducer, it works for about fifty percent of the people who take it.

Cayce Diet—Eliminating Imbalance

For many years, people have been advised to follow a "balanced diet." This is understood to mean that you should eat a wide variety of foods to make sure you are getting the vitamins and minerals your body needs for maximum health. Lacking any other guidelines, this is sound advice. Variety improves the odds that your random selections from one end of the food chain to the other will reap some benefits. This approach was the byword of physicians and nutritionists alike for decades. Unknown to most of them, at the same time Edgar Cayce was peering clairvoyantly into the secrets of food and its passage through the body. He not only provided guidelines for what people should eat and when, but also how meals should be prepared as well as which foods should not be eaten at the same meal. And he even described the proper way to chew food.

The Cayce perspective regarding nutritional balance does not relate to diet alone, but also to bodily functions. The coordination between assimilation and elimination was carefully evaluated during his psychic diagnoses. When imbalance existed between these two activities, remedial directions were given for restoring coordination. This is no small matter, because the two are equal partners in helping to maintain health. If either is not functioning properly, serious complications may develop. You wouldn't think these would have any bearing on longevity, but according to the following comments made to a twenty-eight-year-old man, there is an important connection between these two interrelated activities and our life spans:

There should be a warning to all bodies as to such conditions; for [if] the assimilations and the eliminations would be kept nearer normal in the human family, the days [of life] might be extended to whatever period as was so desired; for the system is builded by the assimilations of that it takes within, and is able to bring resuscitations so long as the eliminations do not hinder. 311-4

The waste products from the foods we digest are essentially toxic. If they remain in the colon longer than normal and are not eliminated, the toxins can find their way back into the system. When you are constipated, the ability to digest foods well is problematic, and the strain on your digestive functions affects your entire body. But it isn't waste alone that causes problems. Foods eaten in wrong combinations or under stressful circumstances can also work to your disadvantage. When you are in a hurry, for instance, you may be prone to cram meals down, as was apparently the case with [311], who was also advised, "Most of all, train self never to bolt the food. Take *time* to assimilate, masticate . . . " (311-4) This was a frequent warning, and reading 808-3 offers this eye-opening assertion: "Bolting food or swallowing it by the use of liquids produces more colds than *any one* activity of a diet!" Digestion begins in the mouth as enzymes in the saliva prepare the food for the stomach. Even milk and water, Cayce stated, should be "chewed" several times to allow them to mix well with the saliva before being swallowed.

It might be said that Cayce did favor one type of "imbalance." He recommended eating largely of the foods that help keep the body in an alkaline condition, and proportionately less of those that make our systems more acidic. But the balance here does not equate with amounts as much as with the effects rendered by acid- and alkaline-producing foods in the body. An alkaline system helps maintain the assimilation-elimination balance. An overacidic system creates complications and makes the body more prone to illness. Excess acids become the breeding ground for colds and flu as well as other conditions. The following comment in reading 1947-4 is echoed by Cayce in numerous commentaries: "Cold germs do not live in an alkaline system! They do breed in any acid or excess of acids of *any* character left in the system."

To that end—alkalinity—he proposed to everyone who needed dietary guidance to rely on large quantities of fruits and vegetables as staples. Fruits and their juices were generally recommended for breakfast, raw vegetables for lunch, and cooked vegetables for the evening meal. A double-barreled benefit comes with fruits and vegetables. While they shift the body's chemistry toward a predominantly alkaline state—with a few exceptions—they also facilitate eliminations.

Fruits and Vegetables

Only twenty percent of the foods we eat daily should be of the acid-producing type, leaving eighty percent alkaline foods from which to select. Fortunately, nature is on our side considering that most food types are alkaline-forming, except for those belonging to the meats and fish category, which fall under the acid-forming group. Nutritionist Simone Gabbay includes a broad list of acid- and alkaline-forming foods in her excellent book, *Nourishing the Body Temple,* which is based on the readings' dietary guidelines. This division is evidence that nature provides us with excellent odds in favor of alkalinity. Most fruits qualify as alkaline-forming, except for blueberries, cranberries, plums, prunes, and sulfured dried fruits. The only vegetables listed as acid-forming are beans, lentils, and garbanzos (chickpeas), though Gabbay indicates these are alkaline-forming when sprouted.

Some people might be surprised to find that citrus fruits are not under the acidic heading. The explanation is that while citrus fruits are acidic in themselves once they are metabolized in our bodies they become alkaline, which is why sipping orange juice, for instance, is helpful in fighting a cold. It should be noted that while overacidity is a condition that invites cold and flu germs to set up house, Cayce added that the body is also prone to colds if it becomes overly alkaline; but that is probably a rare condition for most of us. The readings also advise that adding a teaspoon of lemon juice with the orange juice aids assimilation. For some persons, the ratio was given as four parts orange juice to one part lemon or lime. It was also suggested that when lemon juice is added to water as a drink, which is an excellent alkalizer, adding a little lime juice also helps.

So as it turns out, the body's chemistry has a balance; it's simply maintained by an unequal need for different influences. By eating mainly alkaline-reacting foods and chewing them well, assimilations and eliminations will be "near *normal*," as Cayce put it, and thus years may be added to our life spans—and undoubtedly hours of quality rest to our nights.

The readings also suggest that a good practice is for people to grow some of their own foods. Of course, this addresses the desirability of freshness, as well as the question of alkalinity. In the case of tomatoes that are out of season, for example, Cayce recommended canned tomatoes as suitable if no preservatives have been added. As Gabbay notes, in most cases the tomatoes used for canning are already ripe when harvested and are preserved within hours. Handling and processing "reduces the alkaline-forming values of fruits and vegetables. Harvest-fresh and fully ripe produce is always preferable. When not available, then fruits or veggies naturally preserved or canned in their own juices without additives may be a viable alternative that still provides considerable alkaline-forming properties."

The young man who was told not to bolt his food was also advised to drink plenty of water before and after meals. Many people apparently believe that consuming other liquids, such as carbonated drinks, teas, and juices, suffices in place of water. The readings, however, make it clear that water is a necessary prerequisite in maintaining the assimilation-elimination balance, and it is important to the digestive process. Cayce informed Mr. [311] that when foods reach the stomach, "the stomach becomes a storehouse, or a medicine chest that may create all the elements necessary for proper digestion within the system. If this [stomach] *first* is acted upon by aqua pura, the reactions are more near normal." (311-4) This reading also suggested that when we first arise in the morning it is a good practice is to down one-half to three-quarters of a glass of really warm water—neither too hot nor tepid. Occasionally, a pinch of salt might be added to help flush drosses out of the kidneys. Pure water is a cleansing agent in the body. Six to eight glasses (eight ounces each) were generally recommended as a daily allowance for everyone.

Daily Meals Guidelines

In providing clairvoyant health guidance for individuals, Edgar Cayce sometimes offered detailed suggestions regarding their daily meals, what to eat as well as the best time of day to eat particular foods. The following are examples of the menus he itemized. While he had the advantage of knowing exactly what each of these persons required nutritionally, menus are more or less representative of the emphasis on the acidic-alkaline approach to planning meals.

Reading 3224-2 was for a six-year-old girl, whose parents asked that a daily diet outline be given for the child at the time of the reading "and for the near future":

Mornings—whole grain cereals or citrus fruits, but these never taken at the same meal; rather alternate these, using one on one day and the other the next, and so on. Any form of rice cakes or the like, the yolk of eggs and the like.

Noon—some fresh raw vegetable salad, including many different types. Soups with brown bread, or broths or such.

Evenings—a fairly well coordinated vegetable diet, with three [vegetables] above the ground to one below the ground. Seafood, fowl or lamb; not other types of meats. Gelatine may be prepared with any of the vegetables (as in the salads for the noon meal), or with the milk and cream dishes. These would be well for the body. 3224-2

Reading 1523-17 was for a woman in her mid-thirties who was told the following dietary menus represented only an outline and should not be construed as the only food she should eat:

Mornings—whole grain cereals or citrus fruit juices, though not at the same meal. When using orange juice, combine lime with it. When using grapefruit, combine lemon with it—just a little. Egg, preferably only the yolk, or rice or buckwheat cakes, or toast, or just any one of these, would be well of mornings.

Noons—a raw salad, including tomatoes, radishes, carrots, celery, lettuce, watercress—any or all of these, with a soup or vegetable broth, or seafood or the like.

Evenings—fruits, [such] as cooked apples; potatoes, tomatoes, fish, fowl, lamb, and occasionally beef but not too often.

Keep these as the main part of a well balanced diet. 1523-17

A man in his mid-twenties (135), who was suffering from polio, received a detailed treatment regimen as well as the following menu:

Mornings—only the citrus fruit diet, *changed*, of course, at times, to the hard cereals, whole wheat, whole rice, or corn—as the case may be; but *do not combine* these with the citrus fruits, or have them taken at the same meal! Milk, Ovaltine, or cereal grain extract, may be used as a drink.

Noons—more of the vegetables that are *raw*. These may be made into salads with salad dressings, especially with as much of the olive oil as is palatable and that will be assimilated with the character of foods. This would include lettuce, turnips, cabbage, and all of those that may be used as such. Tomatoes, if they are *ripened on the vine;* otherwise, those that are canned *without* preservative—or especially benzoate of soda. (Do not use such as use that as preservative.) These may be used, especially the juices of same. Any that are palatable, that are raw.

Evenings—flesh may be taken in moderation, but none that does not have the hoof divided and that does not chew the cud. In these, these should not be rendered in other than their *own* fat, and should *not* be in any grease other than their own—whether boiled, fried, or roasted. This will, of course, include breads also. Rye, whole wheat, or it may be mixed. At this meal light wines or malt extracts may be also taken as drinks. 135-1

While the foods recommended here shift the body to a more alkaline state, the combinations of substances also aid assimilation. There is a distinction that is worth noting between assimilation and digestion, although they are not mutually exclusive. Essentially, digestion prepares the food for assimilation as it is chewed and mixed with saliva, then acted on by the gastric acids and enzymes as well as by digestive substances from the gall bladder, liver, and pancreas. When these processes are complete, the converted food particles are absorbed through the stomach wall and distributed throughout the body via the blood and the lymphatic system.

Gabbay observes that the raw-food therapy given in the readings makes sense. "The curative powers of raw vegetables, fruits, and their juices," she states, "derive not only from the abundant vitamins and minerals they contain, but also from the plant enzymes they supply . . . They are organic catalysts necessary for every biochemical reaction in the body."

Food Combinations

Despite the emphasis on vegetables over meats, the readings do not promote a strictly vegetarian diet. This choice was left to individuals to decide for themselves. There are numerous cautionary notes about red meats, however, namely beef and pork, which people were generally discouraged from eating, with the exception of crisp bacon on occasion. The accent on vegetables over red meats seems to be wise advice considering vegetarians have much lower incidences of cancer, diabetes, gallstones, heart disease, and osteoporosis. The wastes that result when beef or pork are eaten can only be burned out of the body by physical exertion, according to the readings. Anyone who is essentially sedentary much of the time is most at risk of eventually suffering the adverse reactions that build up over time. A middle-aged woman who experienced distress in her lower body, which included the sciatic nerves, knees, and feet, received a reading about the condition. Cayce's comments are eye-opening: "These [distresses] began as acute pain, rheumatic or neuritic. They are closer to neuritic-arthritic reactions. This is pork—the effect of same." (3599-1)

Relying on vegetables as the mainstay of our diets will likely increase our odds against developing these ailments. Combining the right foods and avoiding the wrong combinations are also important considerations. As you probably noticed in the meal outlines, Cayce carefully specified eating three vegetables grown above the ground to one grown under the surface. This proportion was given so that combining heavily starchy foods is avoided and assimilations are enhanced. The readings also suggest that it is advisable to refrain from having sweets with foods that are heavy in starch. Sweets with meats, though not particularly encouraged, was mentioned as more acceptable than having sweets and starches at the same meal. The only meats (with the exception of certain small game) that are consistently recommended are modest servings of fish, fowl, or lamb. These are to be cooked only in their own juices by baking, broiling, or roasting, but never frying.

As reading 416-9 explains, assimilations are hampered when starches and proteins are eaten together because they necessitate the use of different gastric juices for digestion. This is also the case when carbohydrates are combined with starchy foods. The specific gastric secretions called into action vary depending on the types of food being digested, and certain secretions work in disparate ways.

In particular, Cayce recommended that meats should not be consumed at the same meal as starches. We should also avoid eating corn, potatoes, rice, or spaghetti, for instance, at the same meal with meat. Two of these together might be okay, but even then they should not be eaten with meat. Thus, by foregoing inappropriate food combinations, we also avoid bringing conflicting gastric secretions into action and, in turn, do not have to suffer the internal consequences. This point is spotlighted in reading 340-32: "There's quite a variation in the reaction in the physical body [to such combinations], especially where intestinal disturbance has caused the greater part of the inflammation through a body . . . " And now we have a clearer idea of what might cause those attention-grabbing episodes of intestinal churning or burning that send us to the medicine cabinet for antacids. According to this reading, the intestines aren't alone; the entire body feels the effects of the disturbance.

Fruits are recommended primarily for breakfast, raw vegetables for lunch, and cooked vegetables for dinner. Citrus fruits, however, are not to be mixed with cereals. Reading 481-1 states that the two together alter the acidity in the stomach, producing detrimental conditions. The reason is that "citrus fruits will act *as* an elimina[nt] when taken alone, but when taken with cereals [they become] as *weight*—rather than as an active force in the gastric forces of the stomach itself."

Various cautions are given in the readings with regard to apples, which should be baked or cooked instead of eaten raw—except for a class of apples referred to as "jenneting." A note to reading 820-2 explains that jenneting is an obsolete word referring to a variety of apple that ripens around St. John's Day, June 24. In another reading (294-182), Cayce named the apples suitable for eating raw: Arkansas Russet, Black Arkansas, Delicious, Jonathan, Oregon Red, and Sheepnose. These were also the types mentioned in connection with the "apple diet," a special regimen the readings recommend as an effective method of cleaning out the intestinal tract. Only raw apples are eaten for three consecutive days. Then on the evening of the third day half a teacup of olive oil is swallowed.[1]

Although vegetables are given thumbs up in the readings, combinations of certain vegetables should be avoided. Some people who received readings from Cayce

---

[1]If you suffer from gallbladder or liver problems, consult your physician before following this diet.

were advised not to mix onions and radishes in the same salad. Exceptions were sometimes allowed if only a small amount of onion was added. Along with the implied caveat of eating three vegetables grown above the ground with each one from below it, the readings also recommend having one leafy vegetable whenever having one of the pod variety. No vegetables should be cooked with either meat or seasoning. If flavoring is required, then salt and a dab of butter can be added when the food is served.

Food Preparation—Ways and Means

A significant aspect of the Cayce dietary guidance involves how foods are best prepared. The readings keep an eye on making sure that foods maintain nutritional integrity, of course, and this relates to the way they are cooked, as well as the means, which received further clairvoyant explanation.

Aluminum: Do you have any aluminum cookware in your kitchen? If so, do yourself a favor and toss it all in the trash—after you take a sledge hammer to these pots and pans so that they cannot be used again. Cayce was firmly opposed to cooking in aluminum utensils, especially when it came to acid-reacting foods such as tomatoes. This is a matter that should not be taken lightly, considering there is a possible link between aluminum poisoning and Alzheimer's disease. Autopsies performed on some patients who suffered from this ailment have revealed the presence of unusual amounts of aluminum in the brain tissues. The best cookware, say the readings, is glass, ceramic, or stainless steel.

Microwave ovens: Microwaves were not yet invented when Cayce was giving his readings, but there is little doubt that his psychic reach would have discovered that this method of cooking presents major complications when it comes to the quality of foods after exposure to these waves. Andrew Weil recommends using the ovens only for heating food. He advises against wrapping foods in plastic, because the waves can drive particles of the plastic into the food. Thus a container suitable for use in the ovens should be used. Gabbay reports on a study that proves the molecular structure of the foods is altered. If the foods are changed, then is it doubtful they are compatible for our assimilative processes. She adds that infant formula manufacturers and physicians tell parents not to use the microwave to warm the formulas. One of the reasons is the chance of uneven heating; another is because of the changes the amino acids undergo. "The fact that microwaving is not recommended for infant foods," Gabbay remarks, "is cause for concern that it may not be a wise choice for older children, adolescents, and adults either."

Pressure cooker: Cooking with pressure was invented about 100 years ago. This method is recommended by the readings, which state that pressure cooking preserves the vitamins and minerals of foods. One person asked specifically if cooking at fifteen pounds of pressure destroys food. Cayce replied that it does not, but explained that it depends on how the foods are prepared and how long before cooking they are harvested, the two factors that determine the food values that remain. Cayce stated further, "As it is so well advertised that coffee loses its value in fifteen to twenty to twenty-five days after being roasted, so do foods or vegetables lose their food value after being gathered—in the same proportion in hours as coffee would in days." (340-31)

Patapar paper: A preferred method of cooking, particularly vegetables, given in the readings is with the use of Patapar paper, a vegetable parchment safe for use with foods. Once a vegetable is prepared and chopped, it is placed in the center of a wet sheet of the parchment. The corners of the paper are lifted and tied together with butcher's string (cotton) to form a small sack. This is placed in a pot of boiling water several inches deep, usually for about fifteen minutes. This allows the vegetable to cook in its own juices. Different vegetables should not be included in the same parchment sack, but they can cook together in the same pot in their own parchment. The juice, needless to say, should not be discarded since it contains many of the nutrients from the food.

Vitamins in the Body

When it comes to vitamin supplements, the readings prefer that people get their nutrition from food alone. Occasionally, of course, exceptions are necessary. Cayce's psychic view was that vitamin-taking—at least in his day—was mostly a fad, except when they were necessary to create a balance in the diet. But a balanced diet precludes the need for extra vitamins.

In reading 2533-6, Cayce's observations are rather pointed and thought-provoking. After prefacing his remarks with the explanation suggesting various combinations of vitamins for treatments, he stated that, " . . . there are only four elements in your body—water, salt, soda and iodine. These are the basic elements, they make all the rest! Each vitamin as a component part of an element is simply a combination of these other influences, given a name mostly for confusion to individuals, by those who would tell you what to do for a price!"

The question was put to Cayce in another reading (2072-9) about the relations that vitamins bear to glands, specifically which vitamins affect which glands. For a moment, the sleeping Cayce balked, saying, "You want a book written on these!" Then he relented and offered the following insights about the functions of certain vitamins:

They [vitamins] are food for same [the glands]. Vitamins are that from which the glands take those necessary influences to supply the energies to enable the varied organs of the body to reproduce themselves. Would it ever be considered that your toenails would be reproduced by the same [gland] as would supply the breast, the head or the face? or that the cuticle would be supplied from the same [source] as would supply the organ of the heart itself? These [building substances] are taken from *glands* that control the assimilated foods, and hence the necessary vitamins in same to supply the various forces for enabling each organ, each functioning of the body to carry on in its creative or generative forces . . .

. . . [Vitamin A] . . . supplies portions to the nerves, to bone, to the brain force itself; not all of this, but this is a part of [what A does].

B and B-1 supply the ability of the energies, or the moving forces of the nerve and of the white blood supply, as well as the white nerve energy in the nerve force itself, the brain [force] itself and the ability of the sympathetic or involuntary reflexes through the body. Now this includes all [the energies], whether you are wiggling your toes or your ears or batting your eye . . . In these [the B vitamins] we have that supplying to the chyle that ability for it to control the influence of fats, which is necessary . . . to carry on the reproducing of the oils that prevent the tenseness in the joints, or that prevent the joints from becoming atrophied or dry, or to creak . . .

In [vitamin C] we find that which supplies the necessary influences to the flexes of every nature throughout the body, whether of a muscular or tendon nature, a heart reaction, or a kidney contraction, or the liver contraction, or the opening or shutting of your mouth . . . These are all supplied by C—not that it is the only supply [for these functions], but [C furnishes] a part of same. It is that from which the structural portions of the body are stored, and drawn upon when it becomes necessary. And when it becomes detrimental, or there is a deficiency of same . . . it is necessary to supply same in such proportions as to aid; else the conditions become such that there are the bad eliminations from the incoordination of the excretory functioning of the alimentary canal, as well as the heart, liver and lungs, through the expelling of those forces that are a part of the structural portion of the body.

G [vitamin B$_2$] supplies the general energies, or the sympathetic forces of the body itself.

These are the principles.

Other vitamins, of course, are mentioned throughout the readings—relative to the nutritional needs of the persons receiving dietary counseling—as well as different minerals, such as calcium, iron, phosphorus, zinc, etc. But the above comments offer a glimpse of the diverse benefits various functions of the body derive from vitamins. The message is obvious—that the body requires right foods in order to function properly.

Foods for Therapy

One of the unique features of the dietary readings is the therapeutic uses that many everyday foods serve. The Cayce approach to healing was always as drug-free as possible. From his clairvoyant viewpoint when diagnosing someone who was physically ailing, a return to balance—healing—was accomplished through the cooperative participation of body, mind, and spirit in association with the divine Source of our existence. It may be said that any illness originates from the misuse of any of these. This is the reason that, along with physical and dietary suggestions, he sometimes saw fit to include psychospiritual advice as well. At the same time, he kept remedial recommendations with regard to food therapies as basic as possible. The following are just a few of the foods mentioned:

The Jerusalem artichoke is one of the basic therapeutic foods discussed by Cayce. A tuber with a texture similar to that of a white potato, it was suggested most often for treatment of diabetes and anemia. It helps the pancreas in regulating glucose levels in the blood. The artichoke is a useful source of insulin when diabetics want to avoid injections. One person was told to eat one tuber a week, or more often, in order to correct "inclinations for the incoordination between . . . the pancreas as related to the kidneys and bladder." (1523-7) Anyone who considers replacing insulin shots with Jerusalem artichokes should do so only under the monitoring eye of a doctor. The amount of the vegetable needed will vary according to the person and the amount of insulin required. One tuber at a time may be eaten either raw or cooked (preferably in Patapar paper); and the recommendation was also to alternate eating the tuber raw and cooked. The skin should be removed, and the artichoke should be eaten with meals.

Watermelon seed tea is an excellent means of purifying the kidneys and bladder, thus improves their function. The tea is made by grinding, cracking, or crushing half an ounce of the seed and letting it steep in a quart of boiling water for twenty minutes. Strain and refrigerate. One person (647-3) was told to take a tablespoonful of the tea twice a day for two or three days, lay off a day or two, and then take again. A pregnant woman (951-7) who asked how to alleviate the pressure on her bladder was instructed to use a teaspoonful of the crushed seed to a pint of boiling water, and to steep it only in a covered enamel or crock container. She was directed to "Take this amount during two days. Then don't take any more for at least three to four days afterwards. Then repeat this." Eating watermelon itself also flushes out the kidneys.

Grape juice is given high marks throughout the physical readings as an internal cleanser. It is also a good source of sugar, Cayce stated without the risk of gaining weight. In fact, the juice is used in a recommended weight-loss regimen. When [3413], who had a bad back, expressed concern about keeping her weight down, Cayce advised her to drink grape juice four times a day, about one-half hour before meals and at bedtime. He explained, "Use three ounces of pure grape juice (such as Welch's) with one ounce of plain water, not carbonated water. This with the [recommended] Sweats or the Baths will keep down the weight as well as remove poisons." (3413-2) Using Concord grapes as a poultice for various purposes was also recommended.

A number of other food therapies are detailed in the readings. For further information, Gabbay's book is an excellent compendium, as is Reilly's *The Edgar Cayce Handbook for Health Through Drugless Therapy*. (See the references section at end of this book.)

Eliminations

The readings give serious consideration to the importance, as already noted, of eliminations. In many of the physical diagnoses, inadequate eliminations were singled out as either a causal or contributing factor in illness. Occasional constipation, of course, plagues virtually everyone at times. But once you are back to a normal schedule, all is well. Isn't it? Maybe, maybe not.

The effects of constipation may remain long after regularity is restored, because some feces may remain caked to the intestinal wall. Several persons, for example, were informed that their shoulder pains—apparently from bursitis—were caused by poisons remaining from poor eliminations. Normal excretory function does not mean all is clear within the colon. This was the primary reason Cayce instructed many people to have a colonic irrigation: Flushing out the colon is the most effective means of assuring a thorough cleaning. As Cayce told one person (3570-1), "One colonic irrigation will be worth about four to six enemas."

Laxatives were sometimes recommended for cleaning the system, as well as for reestablishing regularity. As usual, Cayce's suggestions were at once practical and helpful; and above all, his attention was on the whole person, not merely the condition. A thirty-seven-year-old man was advised to take both a vegetable and a mineral laxative, because it was a good practice to alternate between them: "Have a mineral and again the vegetable compound so there is the better balance kept, and neither will become so necessary or it will not destroy entirely the sphincter activities of the muscular forces of the alimentary canal." (849-76)

Detoxifying the body may seem to have little to do with improving your sleep, but it has a tremendous influence in helping the body to relax. Consider the reply to a fifty-seven-year-old woman (1711-1) who asked what she could do to help her sleep through the night. She was told that purifying her system would "relieve the tensions upon the nervous system in such a way that the functions of the body will bring the normal rest for the body." Stress comes in many forms, as mentioned earlier, including toxins in the system. This is also the apparent reason Cayce added that purification of the body was preferable to taking drugs in order to sleep.

When it comes to specific eliminants, the readings are

eclectic in recommending a variety of substances. The laxatives mentioned range from castor oil to Fletcher's Castoria to syrup of figs to Eno salts (a fruit salt) and others. Usually people were advised to take more than one type. The amounts, frequency, and length of time the laxatives were to be taken depended on the condition and how much cleansing was required. The time could vary from a day to a week or more. A middle-aged woman (379-4) was told not to eat much until she had had "a thorough cleansing of the alimentary canal." Her instructions included taking Fletcher's Castoria and syrup of figs one-half to one hour apart "until there is the *thorough* evacuation."

Poor evacuations, however, are not the sole cause of impurities remaining in the body. Poor eliminations by the kidneys, the lungs, and the skin will also allow the accumulation of drosses, which find their way back into the blood. Thus, for some people, Cayce prescribed hydrotherapy with steam, fume baths, and massage when necessary to help the body expel toxic residues. Let's not forget that there is another important method for the body to assist these organs in throwing off wastes and maintain vitality: exercise. More often than not, even relatively mild exercise gives you the bonus of a good night's sleep.

5

THE REACH OF EXERCISE

If there is such a thing as a natural sleep inducer, it must be exercise. When you are free of worrisome thoughts that burden your mind and your body is free of impurities that cause stress to your joints and nervous system, all you need to add is exercise and you have an almost perfect formula for experiencing peaceful, restoring sleep. Physical activity is one of the elements that contributes balance to your life. The many trillions of cells in the human body form a unified energy field, and the effects of exercise reach all these cells.

Let's review quickly: A mind that dwells on frustrations and problems will be helped by following Cayce's injunction to pray. Even if you have doubts about the efficacy of prayer, it still may help if only because you have turned your thoughts elsewhere. The advice was also given to some people that, if they imagined the body relaxing it would help them release tension. The body with aches and pains can be relieved by heeding the dietary suggestions and cleansing procedures espoused in the readings. These alone are not enough, however, because the body needs to be physically tired—but not exhausted—to sleep well.

For the sake of discussion, exercise may be divided into two broad categories: conditioning and health. Conditioning exercises are done to enhance performance skills in an activity such as dance or sport. Health exercises are self-explanatory and refer to activities aimed at physical well-being and vitality. The reason for making this distinction is to clarify that "no pain, no gain" is a fallacy; it does not apply to physical activity that keeps you healthy.

This is not to suggest that all conditioning workouts are strenuous or that the two categories are mutually exclusive. The distinction is suggested primarily to remind you to follow a course of moderation with regard to exercising, particularly if you are beginning a program after perhaps years of sedentary habits. There is also the matter of individual tolerances, physical potential, previous fitness level, and age to be considered. With regard to advancing, or increasing repetitions of a particular exercise, and the total time spent working out, the older you are, the slower you should progress. After all, what's the hurry? You're not getting in shape for the football season. The most important thing about exercise is settling into the habit and following your routine consistently. And check with your physician before undertaking any exercise program.

A Little Goes a Long Way

When beginning an exercise routine, remember to ease

into it and not push the limit. If you follow a program that involves a series of calisthenics that suggests, for example, beginning with six situps and adding two repetitions every three days, follow the directions. You may know that you can do more than the number stipulated— but don't. By forcing the issue and doing too much too soon, you are likely to tax the body unnecessarily and end up with sore, stiff muscles. If so, you will probably want to lay off the program for a day or two to recuperate, an unnecessary delay. Keep in mind that once you are in the habit of working your muscles, they will cooperate and results will come soon enough. Besides, a little goes a long way, especially when you are just starting out.

In *Ageless Body, Timeless Mind,* endocrinologist Deepak Chopra, who introduced Ayurvedic medicine to America, cites an eye-opening experiment conducted by Swedish psychologist Bengt Saltin. Five young men volunteered to remain in bed around the clock for three weeks to assist Saltin in studying the effects of extended bed rest on the body. The men's physical condition ranged from sedentary to very fit. The shocker came at the end of the three weeks when all of the participants exhibited a drop in aerobic capacity that equated with twenty years of aging. There was another surprising development, as Chopra explains:

> This was a striking finding, but the most fascinating part is that when each subject was allowed to stand up out of bed for five minutes a day, almost the entire loss of function was prevented. They did not have to move around or in any way use their muscles. The simple exposure to a quantum force— gravity—allowed their bodies to remain normal. In a later U.S. study, female runners were tested to see if hard physical exercise helped prevent osteoporo-

sis. The best protection against the disease, some experts feel, is not supplemental calcium or estrogen replacement but building up good bone density in younger years. Since bones get stronger as more weight is brought to bear upon them, long-distance running should increase bone density in the legs by a considerable amount. The application to aging goes beyond osteoporosis, which is an extreme form of bone thinning. Short of acquiring this disorder, old age brings thinner bones in most people, and among the very elderly, hip fractures strike one out of three women and one out of six men.

Studies have proven that exercise indeed increases bone mass. And the benefit is not just bone specific. That is, even if all you do is walk, not only the leg bones increase in density, but your arms bones show a gain as well. As we age, we lose the ability to absorb calcium into our systems, and the bones become thinner. Exercise provides the bonus of stimulating the body's assimilation of calcium and other nutrients.

As for the young men who participated in the Saltin study, over time their physical status would have undoubtedly deteriorated as atrophy set in—along with boredom. But this experiment indicates that even small gestures can bring big gains. The human body is made for activity. Movement is a natural function; it helps increase a sense of well-being and vitality, without which it is difficult to relax or sleep well. Some people who complain of insomnia are in many cases not physically active. There is no question that exercise helps you sleep; it also improves the quality of your nocturnal rest. People who are physically fit and healthy spend more time in the restorative delta stage of sleep.

The advantages of exercise, especially aerobic exercises, are well documented. It is important at any age, and it becomes vital as we get older. By age sixty-five the lungs lose as much as forty percent of their capacity to utilize oxygen. Regular workouts can increase this capacity. There is a tendency, however, for people to become more sedentary with age, thus increasing the risk of age-related illnesses. If you can move your feet, then you can avail yourself of the best exercise of all: walking. The readings often recommend walking in the outdoors as a means for the body to receive exercise.

Take a Walk

A frequently quoted suggestion that issued from Cayce's psychic realm states: "After breakfast work a while, After lunch rest a while, After dinner walk a mile." (470-17) Although only one of the many exercises detailed in the readings, walking was a favorite. When [277] asked which exercise is best, he was told that walking was the better, and also rowing. A woman who suffered from multiple ailments, including arthritis, neuritis, and rheumatism, was advised (1530-2) to exercise daily in the open air. To emphasize the point, Cayce added, "Walking is the best exercise, but this—though—in the *open*, when at all practical."

It has been found that people who walk more than six blocks daily experience one-third fewer sleep disruptions than those who do not get out and stretch their legs. Walkers also have less difficulty falling asleep. Taking a brisk walk and then climbing into bed a short time later, however, may delay your getting to sleep. The body needs a chance to unwind and relax. A brisk walk needs to be completed two or three hours prior to bedtime.

Studies also suggest that whether you walk rapidly or slowly makes little difference in terms of the benefits. In his book, Reilly recommended stride walking, with either long, medium, or short strides. In addition, he suggested that you should walk as fast as possible during the final quarter of a mile in order to work up a good sweat. He observed, "The benefits of brisk walking and striding are increased exercise of the heart, increased oxygen intake, and improved blood circulation." This is a good habit, especially if walking is the only exercise you can arrange to do regularly.

In fact, daily walks are the best way to begin if you are not accustomed to much physical activity, or if circumstances such as a long illness have prevented you from getting adequate exercise. Once you are in the habit of moving your body for a sustained distance as a daily routine, other exercises can be incorporated. Eventually you may be inclined to jog. If so, you should follow Reilly's advice and proceed carefully—after a cardiovascular exam and your doctor's okay.

The best preparation, this physiotherapist believed, is to begin with a series of walks, gradually increasing distance and speed. After a few weeks of speed walking over long distances, you may begin alternating between walking and jogging on your daily outings. As a beginner, you might start out walking three hundred paces, and then jogging slowly with short steps for about a hundred paces, switching back and forth for a half mile. After a few weeks, you may add a hundred jogging steps and decrease your strides by the same number. Reilly calculated that, after six weeks, you will be jogging almost one-half mile. And if you decide to extend the workout another half a mile, he suggested this additional leg of the run should follow the same formula used in the beginning and building up slowly.

Mind What You're Doing

In directing people to exercise, the readings always provided holistic-based guidance. Mind and body are one, and neither is a discrete entity since the one affects the other. Cayce stated that it is well for everybody to exercise in order to counter-balance daily routines. It was also explained in reading 798-1 that the less physical exercise or manual activity people get, the more alkaline-reacting foods they should eat. "*Energies* or activities may burn acids," he said, "but those who lead the sedentary life or the non-active life can't go on sweets or too much starches—but these should be well-balanced."

Throughout the clairvoyant data the maxim is echoed repeatedly that mind is the builder of the physical. In addition, balance requires mind and body to remain in harmony with one another, and with the spirit as well. The participation of the mind during exercise is as important as the activities themselves. Many people use exercise equipment, such as stationary bikes, while reading or watching TV, in effect, treating their workout as a mechanical chore. The mind and body need to be one in purpose for the best results. Reilly was convinced that you should concentrate and give your full attention when exercising, and dispensed this excellent advice:

> Exercises performed absentmindedly with your head full of postmortems or the upcoming problems of the day are not going to do you much good, either in mind or body. Visualize yourself [while exercising] as tall, slim, and flexible, and make a mental picture of the result you want to achieve. This will exercise your involuntary muscle system as well as your voluntary muscles. (This, by the way, is how I have taught paralytics and even paraplegics to regenerate some movement into their bodies . . .)

The workings of the imagination are often thought of as the chimerical musings of an idle mind, a kind of mental frolic at best, and they may be at times. The ability to imagine, however, is a powerful facet of the mind. When applied purposefully, the imagination is used creatively. Albert Einstein said, "Imagination is more important than knowledge." He arrived at his theory of light not by mathematical processes but by imagining himself to be a photon in a stream of light zipping through space, only using math to support his fanciful journey.

The act of exercise must be voluntary and pursued willingly for meaningful results. A positive act of will makes all the difference. As Chopra put it, "When you start to assert control over any bodily process, the effect is holistic. The mind-body system reacts to every single stimulus as a global event; i.e., to stimulate one cell is to stimulate all." This global connection is evidenced by the discovery, mentioned above, that arm bones share in the increased density from exercising the legs. The readings confirm that nothing in our experience surpasses a person's will or determination. As Cayce assured a young man: "For, when the will to do is ever present and not faltered by doubts and fears . . . then does it build, then does it attract that which builds and builds and *is* the constructive force in the experience of all." (416-2)

Chopra made the point that intention stimulates the mind. He cited a remarkable phenomenon exhibited by people who suffer from Parkinson's disease, which is caused by the depletion of dopamine, a vital brain chemical. A patient may take a step or two, but stop as if frozen to the spot. It was discovered that when a line was drawn on the floor and the patient was asked to step over it, "[T]he person will miraculously step over it." This indicates, he said, that the infirmity and inactivity displayed by many old people is merely the result of dormancy: "By renewing their intention to live active, purposeful lives, many elderly people can dramatically improve their motor abilities, strength, agility, and mental responses."

The mind and imagination joined in purpose with the

will and sustained by patience ultimately bring results. A journey implies a destination, movement a purpose. It isn't enough for your doctor to prescribe walking three miles each day; this must be your decision, a positive commitment by the will. Unless you are convinced that it is in your best interest and what you really want to do, then perhaps you should not step over the line at all. Consider Cayce's advice in 457-12 to a woman who asked whether discontinuing situps for several months had been detrimental: "Whenever something is begun and then left off, it be (457-12)

Exercise Programs and Routines

There are many types of exercise programs designed for a variety of goals. Reilly's book details a comprehensive group of exercises for figure and fitness, and includes exercises for all parts of the body, even face and hands. These routines are especially beneficial for your balance, posture, and muscle tone. Many of the movements incorporate exercises given in the Cayce readings, some of which are unique and rarely appear elsewhere. More about these in a moment.

Another excellent program for fitness, particularly for men and women from mid-teens to mid-forties, is *Adult Physical Fitness*, available from the U.S. Government Printing Office. This program assumes that you are beginning without having engaged recently in regular physical activity. For this reason, three general types of exercises are covered—warmup, conditioning, and circulatory activities. Ten orientation exercises—bending and stretching, knee lifting, arm circles, etc.—and a circulatory activity (walking or skipping rope) prepare you for the conditioning exercises.

After a week—or longer if necessary—of gently orienting your muscles, you move on to the conditioning routine, retaining the first six orientation exercises as a warmup for the regular workout. The program calls for five workouts weekly. There are five conditioning levels, each more difficult than those preceding it. You spend at least three weeks at each level before advancing to the next one. A simple "prove-out test" lets you know if you are ready to advance to the next level. There is no requirement at all to advance beyond a level you feel is satisfactory for your purposes, so you can remain at any level indefinitely.

For older adults, *Exercise: A Guide from the National Institute on Aging* is a valuable guide which is available free on request from the Institute (see the resources section at the end of this book). It guides you through exercises to improve balance and endurance, flexibility and strength, as well as providing dietary tips. This book is a fairly comprehensive program that addresses the special needs of the aged and assures that exercise is not only for older adults in the younger part of that age range, but even for those of advanced years. Where there is life there is hope, as the saying goes, and this book reflects an optimistic outlook even for those limited by ailments: "[Exercise] can improve health for older people who already have diseases and disabilities, if it's done on a long-term, regular basis."

Exercise also includes guidance for aerobic activities such as bicycling, swimming, tennis, and walking. It describes various stretching exercises, which are performed sitting, standing, and lying down, and includes directions for using light weights to work the muscles. Throughout the book various helpful hints are included to encourage and keep you on track. The panel of authors adds comments about motivation, including the point that the first month is crucial "to making exercise and physical activity regular, lifelong habits." Anyone over fifty will find valuable guidance in these informative pages.

Exercises from the Readings

Generally, the exercises mentioned most in the Cayce readings involve three primary activities: breathing, calisthenics, and walking. More often than not, the recommendations were case specific and tailored to the individual, though the exercises are helpful to anyone. Cayce also suggested other activities such as bicycling, horseback riding, tennis, and others. Of course, he knew clairvoyantly what resources and facilities were available to the people who received readings. But the three exercises he frequently counseled others to follow require no special accommodations.

While breathing exercises alone are described in the readings, they are usually mentioned in conjunction with stretching movements. Arguably, stretching routines are as important to muscle tone as weight lifting, and perhaps more so when it comes to athletic performance, in which limberness and flexibility are paramount. There is also remedial value to stretching. Cayce told a middle-aged man (4003-1) that stretching would help strengthen his muscles and tendons. This comment was prefaced by the recommendation that "The exercise that we would follow for this body would be the stretching much in the manner as the exercise of the cat or the panther . . . " But without undue strain, it was added. The following stretching-and-breathing exercise was given for a fifty-four-year-old man [470] as a remedy for problems with his sympathetic nervous system. A head-and-neck exercise was mentioned to "relieve those little tensions" associated with conditions in the man's head, eyes, mouth, and teeth. He was advised to do the exercise regularly in the mornings before dressing, to take his time while performing the movements and not to rush:

. . . rise on the toes slowly and raise the arms

easily at the same time directly above the head, pointing straight up. At the same time bend [the] head back just as far as you can. When [you] let down gentle from this you see, we make for giving a better circulation through the whole area from the abdomen, through the diaphragm, through the lungs, head and neck. Then let down, put the head forward just as far as it will come on the chest, then raise again at the top, bend the head to the right as far as it will go down. When rising again, bend the head to the left. Then standing erect, hands on hips, circle the head, roll around to the right two or three times, then straighten self. Again hands off the hip, down gently, rise again, down again, then circle to the opposite side. We will find we will change all of these disturbances through the mouth, head, eyes and the activities of the whole body will be improved. Open your mouth as you go up and down also. 470-37

Obviously, just a little stretching goes a long way; and the fewer clothes you have on while working out, the more freedom of movement you have. Another person was directed in reading 2454-2 to perform the morning exercise of swinging the arms up and down, and also swinging them around in a more or less horizontal motion, allowing the torso to rotate back and around with them. This exercise is intended to "take away the heaviness and the tendency to get tired easily." Stretching the arms above the head, as Cayce explained to [2072], improves assimilation of foods, because they "stimulate the gastric flow and let that eaten have something to float in . . . " (2072-14)

Proper breathing unquestionably is a vital part of physical activity. A fire doesn't get very far without adequate oxygen, and neither does the body. The way to breathe while in a relaxed state is to inhale through the nostrils and exhale through the mouth with the lips barely separated. During periods of exertion, such as running, both the nose and mouth are used for both drawing in and expelling air. The reason Cayce directed people to adopt specific breathing exercises first thing in the morning is that stale air remains in the bottom of the lungs from shallow breathing during the night. Thus, "out with the old air and in with the new" revs the body a bit and gets it ready for the day.

Reilly suggested that while working out you should inhale when straightening your body from a movement and exhale whenever you perform bending movements forward or to the side—but do not exhale when doing backbends. You want to inhale when your body is in the most suitable position to allow the lungs to expand and draw in as much air as possible. It is never a good idea to hold your breath while exerting yourself, because this raises your blood pressure even more. When it comes to flushing out stale morning air, Cayce also described a variation for a twenty-nine-year-old woman who was instructed in the technique of switching from one nostril to the other:

> Of morning, and upon arising especially (and don't sleep too late!)—and before dressing, so that the clothing is loose or the fewer [you have on] the better—standing erect before an open window, breathe deeply; gradually raising hands *above* the head, and then with the circular motion of the body from the hips bend forward; breathing *in* (and through the nostrils) as the body rises on the toes— breathing very deep; *exhaling suddenly* through the *mouth; not* through the nasal passages. Take these for five to six minutes. Then as these progress, gradually *close* one of the nostrils (even if it's necessary to

use the hand—but if it is closed with the left hand, raise the right hand; and when closing the right nostril with the right hand, then raise the left hand) *as* the breathing *in* is accomplished. Rise, and [then do] the circular motion of the body from the hips, and [the] bending forward; *expelling* as the body reaches the lowest level in the bending towards the floor (expelling through the mouth, suddenly). See?

Then of an evening, just before retiring—with the [body prone, facing the floor and] feet braced against the wall, circle the torso by resting on the hands. Raise and lower the body not merely by the hands but more from the torso, and with more of a circular motion of the pelvic organs to strengthen the muscular forces of the abdomen. Not such an activity as to cause strain, but a gentle, circular motion to the right two to three times, and then [as many times] to the left. 1523-2

As a rule, the readings favored standing exercises in the morning and floor exercises in the evening. This was not a hard and fast rule, however. It was suggested in reading 4462-1 that performing situps first thing in the mornings would aid the lungs and blood supply and invigorate the muscles. The situps were to be followed by five or ten minutes of exercising the arms and limbs. The purpose of morning vertical exercises, as just shown, is to pump fresh oxygen into the body, while evening horizontal exercise is to counteract the effects of being upright all day by balancing circulation throughout the body.

Common Sense

As with all things human, exercise is a highly individual matter. Just as people have different nutritional requirements, so it is with physical activity. This is mentioned in particular to dissuade you from any tendency to make fruitless comparisons between your physical activities and those of others. If your neighbor takes a daily two-mile walk and is obviously full of vitality, this should not prompt you to shorten your three-mile walk—or vice versa—if you feel your distance is right for your purposes. This is another reason to keep your mind tuned to what you are doing. You want to be aware of your body's response. The distance you walk, or the number of repetitions performed during a given exercise, is less important than the effect. When beginning a routine, the rate of progress and the benefits that accrue also vary with individuals. So trust your deeper instincts.

Another point to keep in mind is that most people do well with exercise without a personal instructor. If you have special needs that must be taken into consideration relative to exercise, you may want to consult with a professional fitness advisor. Be aware, however, that anyone may claim to be a professional since no certification standards are required to justify the title. The best approach is to find a qualified physical therapist or other professional trained in sports medicine. You may want to contact the American College of Sports Medicine for a list of health professionals nearest you. (See the resources section at the end of this book.)

Meanwhile, if you are not physically active or otherwise not getting enough exercise, make it a priority. You will feel better and certainly sleep better. At the same time, keep in mind this Cayce comment:

"Exercise is wonderful, and necessary—and little or few take as much as is needed, in a systematic manner. Use common sense. Use discretion." (283-1)

6

PRISMS OF THE MIND

There is no doubt that animals sleep, but while humans generally require an average of eight hours' sleep a night, mammals exhibit a wide variation in the amount of time spent snoozing. Among all mammals, the total number of hours spent sleeping reveals striking contrasts. For example, bats are perennial sleepyheads and spend almost twenty hours asleep, but giraffes grab only about two hours of shut-eye. Your everyday domestic cat outsleeps you by quite a bit, clocking as many as twelve hours, though the mighty lion nestles in for thirteen and one-half hours. The baboon, aping humans it seems, uses nine hours each night.

Some mammals have made unusual adaptations for sleep. For example, cattle sleep with their eyes open. Not only do dolphins and porpoises possess the unique ability to doze while cruising beneath the sea, they sleep with only half of their brains. Apparently the other half remains alert so that they will periodically remember to come up for air. Animals also demonstrate REM and non-REM sleep. But whether their sleep is short or long, other creatures may have an advantage over us in that they do not seem to be plagued by a mind that clings to concerns and difficulties of the day. They show no signs of being tormented by their own thoughts. That habit is reserved for us humans.

Indeed, it is a fascinating fact that our thoughts are not necessarily our best friends. And the stream of our reflections at times may thunder wildly like a runaway train barreling along the tracks of our emotions. More often than not, the emotions are negative reactions and attitudes, which evoke all-too-familiar images that we have projected repeatedly onto the screens of our minds. You might think your consciousness would say, *Enough of this internal dialog, let's go to sleep.* But the mind obviously does not work like that. It processes only what you feed it. If you insist on revisiting old grudges and thoughts of revenge, the mind is at your service. In turn, your thoughts will arouse associated emotions, and you will again experience the same anger you experienced from the actual event. The mind does not automatically discern between the real and the imagined; they are both the same. As disconcerting as it may be to lie in bed unable to sleep because your mind will not settle down, why fault the mind for the problems churning through it? True, they are real concerns, these fretful memories and imaginings, thus are obviously valid or you would not be rehashing them. Or is it that, like a kaleidoscope, your mental faculties are merely reflecting worrisome conditions that the mind has nothing to do with? This might seem to be the case.

Nevertheless, when the mind is besieged by unsettling

thoughts and cannot accept the cloak of sleep, the ramifications of the phenomenon need to be explored. People
sometimes say they understand their own minds. Usually they mean they are clear about their likes and dis-
likes, their biases and preferences. The mind in itself is
much more than a cognitive inventory of your personal
idiosyncrasies. But understanding it and the many facets
associated with its function is like confronting an enigma
wrapped inside a mystery.

In Search of the Mind

The elusive nature of mind has challenged philosophers for ages. It was not until the seventeenth century,
however, that the subject generated much discussion.
This resulted from the body-mind ruminations of René
Descartes, who wondered whether the mind, or consciousness, is something different from matter and considered whether consciousness is physical or nonphysical.
English philosopher John Locke and others proposed that
consciousness is produced by physical sensations as well
as by the data received through them.

Various psychologists, including Freud, also took on
the quest to establish the nature of consciousness. Then
early in the twentieth century psychologist John Watson,
leading the behaviorism movement, dismissed any need
for terms such as mind and consciousness. This view steered
psychology back to an objective study of the subject, relying on measured responses to stimuli to explain behavior.
After all, science cannot study what cannot be observed.

Consciousness did not receive much attention for several more decades. There was a renewal of interest in
hypnosis, along with an increasing curiosity about
dreams and meditation. A revival of things spiritual, not
merely secular, seems to have made us more receptive to
practices and disciplines from Eastern cultures. Medita-

tion, which Cayce had been recommending in his psychic commentaries for half a century, established itself in America. Thus mind regained the spotlight despite having been upstaged for a time by the view that we mortals are hardly more than organic machines.

It is convenient, and perhaps simplistic, to assume that mind is simply the collateral effect from electrochemical processes in the brain. Yet, important issues persist regarding the mind and consciousness. In *Quantum Healing*, Deepak Chopra cites a heart disease study conducted in the 1970s. Groups of rabbits were fed very toxic, high-cholesterol foods to block the animals' arteries. Results appeared consistently in all the groups but one, which unaccountably showed sixty percent fewer symptoms. The physiology of the rabbits did not explain this discrepancy. Then it was found that the student responsible for tending this particular group liked to fondle and stroke them, holding each rabbit for a few minutes prior to feeding. This contact apparently helped the rabbits overcome the effects of the toxic diet. Follow-up experiments showed similar results. Chopra observes that "the mechanism that causes such immunity is quite unknown—it is baffling to think that evolution has built into the rabbit mind an immune response that needs to be triggered by human cuddling." He states further:

> There is even a possibility, many doctors would contend, that the mind is a fiction, medically speaking. When we think that it is sick, what is really sick is the brain. By this logic, the classical mental disorders—depression, schizophrenia, and psychosis—are actually brain disorders. This logic has obvious inadequacies: it is like saying that car wrecks should be blamed on automobiles. But the brain, being a physical organ that can be weighed and dissected, makes medicine feel more secure than does the

mind, which has proved impossible to define after many centuries of introspection and analysis. Doctors are quite happy not to be called upon as philosophers.

From a strictly holistic standpoint, of course, the brain-mind connection is a two-way street. This means the cause of a mental disorder may originate in either one or the other. While mind/consciousness is currently beyond the grasp of science and medicine, it is a tenable subject for metaphysics. When Descartes postulated, *Cogito, ergo sum*—"I think, therefore I am"—it was an idea related to his contention that God exists, that He created two classes of things: minds and bodies as two distinct substances. The philosopher's views are not unlike those presented by the Cayce readings.

Metaphysics of Mind

The explanation of mind given in the readings is challenging and entails many absorbing implications. To better understand the nature of this mental faculty as discussed by Cayce, we will go back in time to the creation of the world as revealed by the readings. The following is only a brief sketch of the extensive commentary in the 262 series of readings.

When God created souls, He gave each of us two attributes: mind and will. Without sentience and choice, we would be nothing more than robots; the Creator, however, wanted companions, not puppets. Thus we came into our divine estate, conscious of ourselves as individual souls and of our relationship to the Creator. There were also other, denser bodies that were not like us. The planets, stars, and other things material possessed slower vibrations; and in our natal beginning as souls they must have been curious and fascinating.

By poking around, as it were, we discovered that our finer vibrations could easily penetrate and mesh with those of material bodies, plants, and animals. We continued to experiment, entering and leaving these forms at will, even altering their physical characteristics. Then, over time, something went amiss. We obviously had no idea what we were doing, because our obsession with the material world backfired, and we assumed physical bodies, thus became trapped in the earth plane, locked into the cycles of physical life and death.

All souls were not tempted, thus did not "fall" into matter. For those of us who succumbed to the pull of physical urges, matters turned even worse. We were able for a time, despite the distractions of our physical bodies, to remain aware of our divine origin, with full knowledge of who we truly are and our relationship to God, but then our minds became divided, as evidenced by the split brain, its separate hemispheres with their different functions. Incidentally, it may well be that this division is allegorized by the Old Testament account of Cain killing his brother Abel. Cain represents the left brain, with its ego and self-indulgent urges, while Abel is the right brain that seeks to maintain contact with God. So it was that we were born into a preoccupation with the physical and died in spiritual awareness.

We should consider that it was not until we became crystallized forms that our free wills were truly challenged as a vital force in determining our destinies. In reading 3744-2, Cayce defined mind as the active force within animate objects, and in the image of the Creator. Then he made this riveting statement: "Mind is the factor that is in direct opposition of will." From this contrast, it may be surmised that mind and will are to be one in purpose, not in conflict. In its relationship to will and body, mind is the mediator. As the psychic explained further: "Mind being and is the factor governing the con-

tention, or the interlaying space, if you please, between
the physical to the soul, and the soul to the spirit forces
within the individual or animate forces."

When Cayce stated that mind is the builder, he often
added that it may produce either crimes or miracles, depending on the way it is used. In reading 826-11, he
added another point in saying, "Mind is the builder, being both the spiritual and material; and the consciousness of same reaches man only in his awareness of his
consciousness through the senses of his physical being."
Here in the third dimension, the conscious mind is our
immediate resource through which we may connect to
higher states of awareness. There are three dimensions of
mind: the conscious, the subconscious, and the superconscious. Our subconscious is the soul's conscious mind,
and the superconscious is the soul's subconscious. The
relationship of our conscious to the subconscious is like
that of the subconscious to the superconscious. The mind
and will of us mortals present dual challenges, as indicated in the following statement Cayce made when asked
to explain what was meant by the mind being in direct
opposition to will:

> We have many phases of mind. We have the mind
> of the spirit consciousness, of the physical sub-con-
> scious, or soul. We have the mind of the physical
> body, through which any or all of these may mani-
> fest. The will [is] that active principle against which
> such manifestations respond. Hence [it is in] direct
> opposition to mind action. This, we find then, refers
> to the condition in the material world, will, see? The
> will in the spiritual plane, or spirit consciousness
> (not spirit entity) being the creation of that mani-
> fested in the earth plane. Hence the different condi-
> tions in will's manifesting and in how will [is in]
> opposition to the mind forces.

. . . Knowledge comes through the senses in the physical body to the conscious mind. The subconscious has the storing of the knowledge of given conditions; when the consciousness receives through the sense that knowledge, the will [is] the action against the incentives set forth. 900-21

It should be clear from this material that mind is something apart from the brain. The readings make this assertion, in fact, and add in reading 826-11 that mind uses brain. In the brain and the body, however, a prism effect occurs and the forces of the mind are directed by different urges and activities. The mind as expressed in the physical world is like a house divided against itself. In *The History and Power of the Mind,* occult lecturer Richard Ingalese explained it this way at the dawn of the twentieth century: "Consciousness is limited in its manifestation by the medium or media through which it manifests." Left to its own devices, the conscious mind will always follow self-serving urges. Despite the finite use that mind serves through the left brain, it remains essentially transcendent, because it is in essence divine. Fortunately, the brain does not tell the whole story of mind; if it did, then thoughts could hardly generate things. Thoughts sustained by mind can become actualized. Ingalese describes the process this way:

Divine mind is precisely analogous to a sensitive plate and each human thought makes a picture on that plate. By thought you make the exposure, and the thing pictured will in time become your own, for you are attached to your creations and time develops the picture for you. If you hold the image you have made long enough, you will get a perfect picture; if you think idly, then you have made what the photographers would call an underexposure and the picture is not full, clear and perfect, and many of the details are left out; but by holding the picture firmly and strongly, you make it a permanency and then it is yours, for thoughts become things.

Mental pictures are first mental things, but after a time they become physical things or draw physical things to them, for the great Consciousness gives back to us precisely what we send into it. It gives to us whatever we ask of it, and our ignorance in making demands will be no protection to us. The only way that evolution can go on is by Divine Mind granting every request that we persistently make; it is in this way we gain wisdom through experience.

In addition, this process helps clarify the spiritual truth Jesus taught: "Judge not that ye be not judged." (Matthew 7:1) Divine mind is nondiscriminating, thus does not qualify the image we project, nor make any determination as to whether the image is in our best interest. "For with what judgment ye judge, ye shall be judged; and with what measure ye mete, it shall be measured to you again." (Matthew 7:2) In modern vernacular: What you see is what you get—in the sense that your perceptions reveal as much about you as what you perceive.

As individualized entities of the Whole, the Oneness, we get as good as we give—or as bad. Remove the distorting prisms that give the illusion of separateness, and we experience the One Consciousness. In *The Golden Thread of Oneness*, Jon Robertson observes, "Consciousness, basically, is *everything*. It is the eternal flame of awareness, and it is also our eternal presence in the endless 'now.' The flame does not go out, not even when we are asleep or when our bodies die." Nor do the consequences of our thoughts and actions die with us. As part of the One, we are accountable—not necessarily accountable with regard to particulars but to the spirit behind our thoughts and actions. The spirit in which we live continually revisits us, whether from day to day, from year to year, or from one lifetime to another. As Cayce reminded us: We meet ourselves. And considering the spirit in which many of us live—our mean-spirited thoughts and unforgiving attitudes—it is amazing we get any sleep at all.

Reading 2067-3 defines sleep as a sense that is needed for the physical body to recuperate. While asleep we "draw from the mental and spiritual powers or forces that are held as the ideals of the body." We are cautioned not to think of the body as an incidental machine or to imagine that whatever happens to us is merely chance. All is predicated on law, and what happens to us while sleeping depends on what we have thought, which reflects the ideals we embrace. It is a fact that there are people who, because of what they think and how they live, gain strength and vitality from sleep. On the other hand, there are those who may feel dejected or ill after sleeping. Cayce stresses that, in either case, this is in accordance with the law behind our existence.

This takes us to the matter of purpose, and of our relationship to the Whole and to one another. Reading 826-11 states that we are physical, mental, and spiritual entities. The spiritual is the portion that is everlasting; it is also a part of all it has ever applied in its mental experiences during the soul's journey. Where, Cayce asked rhetorically, does this spirit body come from? The spirit is of the universal consciousness, or God, who is the First Cause, and the spirit of a person is a portion of the First Cause. As we manifest our purpose in the material world, in physical consciousness, the more we grow in awareness of the relationship of our mental and physical bodies to the infinite God-consciousness.

Our purpose, we are told, is to know our relationship to the Creator—for each entity to know itself to be an individual and also a part of the Whole, the full recognition of which constitutes our purpose and reason for being. Complications arise, however, whenever we allow ourselves to be distracted, "when there is such a diffusion of consciousness as to change, alter or create a direction . . . [that causes an entity] to waver . . . from its purpose for being in a consciousness, it loses its individual identity." (826-11) In short, when we forfeit our purpose, there is no purpose for our being; thus, we may ultimately cease to exist at all.

In the context of mind as the builder, as cited earlier, it is through the senses that we may be aware that mind is both spiritual and material. The sentient quality referred to here includes not merely the mundane senses, but also the endocrine glands, which serve as spiritual contact points in the body in addition to their glandular activities. The senses are vital influences, and it is important just how we allow them to be directed, as Cayce comments:

> Then indeed do the senses take *on* an activity in which they may be directed in that awareness, that consciousness of the spiritual self as well as in the physical indulgences or appetites or activities that become as a portion of the selfish nature of the individual or entity.
>
> It behooves the entity first in its premise then to know, to conceive, to imagine, to become aware of that which is its ideal . . .
>
> These meditated upon then, these kept in the ways that ye know. It is not then that ye *know* as a physical consciousness, but that ye *apply* of good, of that which *is* of God, that makes ye know that consciousness of His walks with thee.
>
> For thy physical self may only see the reflection of good, while thy spiritual self may *be* that good in the

activities of thy fellow man in such measures that ye bring—what?

Ever, *ever*, the fruits of the Spirit in their awareness; longsuffering, brotherly love, patience, kindness, gentleness, *hope* and faith!

If ye in thy activities in any manner with thy fellow man destroy these in the minds, in the heart of thy fellow man, ye are not only slipping but ye have taken hold on the path of destruction.

Then so love, so act, so *think* that others *seeing* thy good works, thy hopes that ye bring, thy faith that ye manifest, thy patience that ye show, may *also* glorify Him.

For that cause, for that purpose ye entered into the materiality in the present. 826 -11

All of us have a great deal of responsibility in following the purpose of our existence, which clearly is spiritual even in the physical world. To live other than in accordance with the purpose for our being created as individualized expressions of the Whole is ultimately self-destructive. In the material world, warring within ourselves is the first sign that something is seriously wrong, and a house divided against itself does not sleep well.

The Spiritual Path to Sleep

In *Ageless Body, Timeless Mind*, Chopra observes that "Your life can be only as free as your perception of it." Perception is the key word here. The way you perceive yourself, your circumstances, and your relationships is crucial. Too often, however, human perception takes its cues from limited information and preconceived notions. Chopra reviews a checklist he uses when he finds himself in disagreement with another person and recommends these steps to his readers. When you are in conflict with someone it helps to realize, first of all, that yours is only one view, to concede both may be valid, and to keep in mind your view is limited. At the same time, note any tension in your body, which is a sign you may be holding too adamantly to your position. Then consider matters from a new perspective, and you will see things a little differently. Finally, question your interpretation to determine whether it still seems valid. Chopra offers an especially helpful tip in stating that you should concentrate on the process, not the outcome, and not concern yourself with "how something *has* to turn out."

This self-inventory approach is one that Edgar Cayce would certainly approve. He often urged individuals to "watch self pass by." Once you get an objective grip on your inner responses, your views and reactions shift to a more reasonable outlook, and you develop the habit of easing back on the throttle of your emotions when a disagreement arises between you and another person. Entrenching your position, on the other hand, only aggravates the conflict. Besides, what's more important, your point of view or peace of mind—being right or being relaxed?

While Chopra's suggestions are aimed at dealing with stressful situations, to apply them is to adopt a constructive attitude, one that allows the fruits of the spirit to flourish within yourself and others. In the reading excerpt above, we are told that cultivating these fruits is in accord with our spiritual purpose. As one young man was advised in 416-2, "Speak kindly, speak in convincing ways and manners of that which is thine own experience. For, each soul must apply—especially spiritual, but also mental—truths in its own experience." The fruits are indeed the demonstration of the ideal truths of the spirit. Study Chopra's steps in ameliorating a conflict as a starting point. He adds, however, that the approach first requires some preparation, so he suggests the following exercise, which you can use in connection with someone who has hurt your feelings deeply in the past and whom you have a hard time forgiving:

1. I feel hurt, but that doesn't mean the other person was bad or meant to hurt me. He doesn't know my entire past, and I don't know his. There's always another side to the story, despite my hurt.

2. I've been hurt like this before, and therefore maybe I was too quick to judge this incident. I need to see each thing as it is.

3. I don't need to see myself as a victim here. When was the last time I was on the other side of the same situation? Didn't I feel pretty caught up in my own motives? Did I give any more importance to the other person's hurt than mine was given this time?

4. Let me forget my feelings for a second. How did that other person feel? Perhaps he just lost control or was too wrapped up in his own world to notice my hurt.

5. This incident can help me. I don't really care about blaming this person or getting back. I want to find out the kinds of things that create threat in me. The more I think about it, the more I see this as an opportunity to take responsibility for my feelings. That makes it easier for me to forgive, since anyone who teaches me something about myself deserves my thanks.

When you begin to get into the habit of consciously and carefully examining your old interpretations in this way, you create a space for spontaneous moments of freedom. These are the moments when your old mindset clears in a flash of insight. With that flash comes a sense of revelation, because you are looking into reality itself, not a reflection of your past. All the most valuable things in life—love, compassion, beauty, forgiveness, inspiration—must come to us spontaneously. We can only prepare the way for them (a spiritual friend of mine calls this "punching a hole into the fourth dimension").

This exercise is an excellent way to help free your mind from the tendency of "cognitive distortions" discussed in an earlier chapter. The conscious mind simply does not see the entire pattern of dynamics that shapes its human circumstances. Thus, it is sound advice—and the first step toward wisdom—to question your assumptions and automatic responses, as well as to review and modify them realistically. By taking a more reasonable, open-minded attitude toward your own views, you will better understand the views of others. As you develop more flexible responses to opposing points of view, you will discover others are more flexible also. And by dealing with people in the right spirit, as revealed by your attitude, you nourish and touch their spirits. This is in accord with your purpose and, as Cayce indicated, it is law. In *As a Man Thinketh*, James Allen reminds us that "Law, not confusion, is the dominating principle in the universe . . . " It is in the context of this principle that Allen explains in no uncertain terms—which, it goes without saying, also apply to a woman:

A man only begins to be a man when he ceases to whine and revile, and commences to search for the hidden justice which regulates his life. And as he adapts his mind to that regulating factor, he ceases to accuse others as the cause of his condition, and builds himself up in strong and noble thoughts; ceases to kick against circumstances, but begins to *use* them as aids to his more rapid progress, and as a means of discovering the hidden powers and possibilities within himself.

Confusion, of course, is possible because of the dual nature of our minds, because confusion originates only in our minds. In the body, the right brain is inclined to spiritual impulses, while the left is the minion of the physical urges. If this were not the case, then we would not be burdened with a conscience, which is simply the still, small voice of the soul trying to get a word in edgewise through the clatter and clutter of the conscious mind.

Most of us tend to think that the opposite of love is hate, but Cayce stated that its opposite is indifference. Love is attachment, the other detachment. Hatred, however, is also attachment in that the emotions are just as wrapped up in the other, except in a hostile way. To forgive someone for a minor injury to the ego is one thing, but some people have difficulty letting go of more serious wrongs committed against them. Decades after the outrage, they only have to recall the person and those long-ago emotions begin to seethe. Actually, they are not old emotions at all. The memory may be decades old, but the emotions are quite contemporary and just as painful as if the situation had just occurred. People who have a terrible wrong branded into their minds are often heard to say, "I'll never forgive . . . " It is an unfortunate decision, despite the injustice they have suffered.

For those who are tired of lugging around old grudges and seek to forgive and forget, there is a way. This approach involves a unique prayer aimed at releasing your rancorous attachment to someone who has deeply wronged you. It is a method of prayer originated by metaphysical writer Everett Irion, who called it "The Forty-Day Prayer." He first published the prayer in the early 1980s in his column, which appeared in *Venture*

Inward magazine. Afterward he received numerous letters of appreciation from people who discussed how they had been helped by the prayer.

This is a spirit-to-spirit prayer, as it were, because you direct your statement to the other person—not, however, in person. You then address the prayer to yourself, your own spirit. The wording of the prayer does not have to be verbatim as shown here, as long as the same meaning and intent are conveyed. After all, prayers are not merely based on words. Here is the wording:

> **[Person's name (full name, if known)]** I am praying to you. Please forgive me for everything I have ever done to you. Thank you, **[Name of person]**, for everything you have ever done to me.

Remember, to say the prayer twice: first using the person's name, and second using your own name. Here are other important points to keep in mind:

- Repeat the prayer once each day, preferably at about the same time, for forty days.
- If at any point you forget and skip a day, begin again at day one and continue until forty consecutive days have been covered without missing a day.
- If you find yourself having negative thoughts about the person, repeat the prayer at that time. Avoid anticipating the results and thinking of how *you* want matters to turn out.
- Tell no one you are using the prayer.
- It makes no difference whether the person is alive or dead.

Using this prayer makes good sense, and especially spiritual sense. In his trance state, Cayce found no difficulty with anger itself, but warned others against allowing it to become a destructive influence. Ms. [1551] was told that she often allowed an unkind word to grow and magnify into a personal insult; she was cautioned that this "will become as a separating thing from those with whom there is not only duty, not only obligations because of associations and relations. But do not let *anger* be thy *destructive* principle! Be mad, yes—but sin not!" (1551-2) A young man was informed in reading 1005-17 that "To worry or to become cross and antagonistic creates poisons that are already in excess [in your body]. Smile even though it takes the hide off, even when you are cross—this will be very much better [than worry]."

Holding on to anger and allowing hostile emotions to play through your mind are poisonous to your physical and mental health, and demeaning to your spirit. Once the cobwebs are cleaned out of the attic of the mind and emotions and memories, sleep comes easily, because it is then undisturbed by inner states of dis-ease. Your conscience will be clear, and your dreams will lift your spirit—and that is who you really are.

7

FOLLOW YOUR DREAMS

The quest for understanding sleep continues. Researchers have assembled a great deal of information, and they are continually discovering new facts. It has been found, for instance, that when you learn a new skill, your ability improves only after a good sleep of at least six hours. The brain apparently uses these hours to register the information in its memory banks. Scientists have explored brainwave patterns, studied the symptoms of sleep loss, and determined that sleep is necessary, although a comprehensive definition remains elusive.

A generally accepted explanation is given by Chopra (*Restful Sleep*), who defines sleep as "a distinct state of mind and body in which the body is deeply at rest, the metabolism is lowered, and the mind becomes unconscious to the outside world." He qualifies this observation by adding that the sleeping mind is not entirely unconscious and mentions that during dreams the brain works harder than when awake. As mentioned earlier, brain-wave measurements show that this is particularly true during the rapid-eye-movement (REM) stage of sleep, which has been equated with dreaming.

These darting eye movements, which occur periodically during sleep, were first noted in 1953, and subsequent research established REM as the dream stage. Yet this does not prove out in every case. Although eighty percent of people roused from REM sleep report dreams, a smaller percentage also recall dreams when awakened from non-REM sleep. Often the non-REM dreamers, however, are likely to recall their dreams more as thoughts in the mode of the waking state.

Generally dreaming is looked upon as a process in the brain, an electrical activity as the brain recoups during sleep. There is speculation that dreams relate to waking urges, desires, needs, etc. Dreaming and dreams are also studied by researchers, who have found that scenes with visual images are recalled eighty percent of the time. It may be that the pictorial displays are those that cause REM for the fact that they are visual and thus readily remembered for the same reason. In most instances, the settings of dreams are in everyday surroundings, although many take on an unreal quality, most likely because the dream world defies the laws of time and space. Transitions from one place to another can happen instantly; or you are looking at a feather in your hand and suddenly it's a knife, or you are simultaneously in two separate scenes in different locales.

Understandably, your dreams in most cases are populated with people you know, either acquaintances or, to a lesser extent, family members. You may awaken on occasion with the awed impression that you were actually where the dream took place and talked to the people in your dream. At any rate, dreams are presumed to be the product of the sleep state. We separate them from fantasy and daydreaming, which are products of the waking mind. Yet, do dreams belong only to the domain of sleep? In *A New Model of the Universe*, P.D. Ouspensky, mathematician, journalist, and formidable thinker, proposes that we dream all the time, even when awake, although we may not be aware it:

> . . . I came to the conclusion that dreams can be observed while awake. It is not at all necessary to be asleep in order to observe dreams. Dreams never stop. We do not notice them in a waking state, amidst the continuous flow of visual, auditory, and other sensations, for the same reason for which we do not see stars in the light of the sun. But just as we can see the stars from the bottom of a deep well, so we can see dreams which go on in us if, even for a short time, we isolate ourselves whether accidentally or intentionally, from the inflow of external impressions. It is not easy to explain how this is to be done. Concentration upon one idea cannot produce this isolation. An arrest of the current of usual thoughts and mental images is necessary. It is necessary to achieve for a short period "consciousness without thought." When this consciousness comes dream images begin slowly to emerge through the usual sensations, and with astonishment you suddenly see yourself surrounded by a strange world of shadows, mood, conversations, sounds, pictures. And you understand then that this world is always in you, that it never disappears.

Ouspensky makes it clear that he is referring to his own experiences, and when he was in the state of "consciousness without thought," there was a sense of *this has happened before.* The Cayce readings explain that here in the third dimension time does not exist as we perceive it, and that all time is one time. So, we may assume that Ouspensky managed to punch a hole through the time barrier or at least to experience a dimension of consciousness in time that we are normally unaware of while in the full waking state. The experience he describes is somewhat akin to going into the meditative state. Practiced meditators, however, move through the "strange world of shadows" and into the blank stillness, the realm of superconsciousness, where there are no distractions. It is probably reasonable to assume that Ouspensky experienced what is referred to as lucid dreaming, a type of dreaming that allows the sleeper to consciously observe or even participate in the process and control the dream scenario.

Cayce confirmed the idea of dreams going on perpetually. Even while we are awake, the soul mind tries to give us guidance. As for whether we are tuned in to the guidance is a matter the psychic likened to our association with others. Just as we do not always desire to be in someone's company, neither do we always remain open to dreams or the soul's influence. It should be noted that Cayce made no distinction between visions and dreams. In our waking state, we may experience intuitive flashes, which is another name for extrasensory perception, but the source is the same.

While the readings endorse the notion of sleep as necessary for the body to recuperate, they reach further into the human condition by stating that sleep is a sense that allows us to draw from the mental and spiritual forces those influences that we hold as ideals. In this connection, as already noted, Cayce commented that there are persons who gain strength and power during sleep, while others wake up feeling ill or dejected. In reading 2067-3 he admonished a middle-aged woman to take time for sleep, because it is the exercising of a faculty and is intended as a portion of each soul's experience:

> It is as but the shadow of life, or lives, or experiences [in the earth], as each day of an experience is a part of the whole that is being builded by an entity, a soul. And each night is as but a period of putting away, storing up into the superconscious or the unconsciousness of the soul itself. 2067-3

This interaction is part of the process of reaping what we sow. Our thoughts, actions, and attitudes come home to roost, for we are accountable within our own souls for all that we are. It is the reconciling of cause and effect that originates from the First Cause, or God. This principle is also an integral function of our dreams. But before taking a closer look at what the readings say about sleep and dreams, let's look at some related dynamics of our human existence as explained by the psychic information.

You Are Here

Earlier, we took a quick look at the account of how we earthbound souls ended up here in the material world. And here we are, self-exiled by our own wills and captives of physical urges that distract us from the full realization of our existence, of our true purpose for being. Thus, we are body, mind, and spirit in a three-dimensional setting. It is in this arena that our purpose still holds, and we live, as Cayce asserted, in time, space, and patience. These three together are the context in which we experience our lifetimes in the earth. They are the three dimensions of consciousness. As one reading explains:

> Each soul, each entity makes upon time and

space—through patience recording same—that as may be indeed the record of the intent and purposes, as well as the material manifestations of the entity through its sojourns in materiality. 1681-1

Patience has a special meaning in the metaphysical discourses. Cayce referred to it as persistent, active patience, not simply passive. Patience is expressive of attitude, and reveals our finite awareness of the spiritual forces behind objective reality as our intents and purposes are recorded upon time and space. Numerous readings echo the view that patience is a lesson each of us must learn here in the earth. In reading 1554-3 we are given to understand that "in Patience then does man become more and more aware *of* the continuity of life, of his soul being a portion of the Whole; Patience being the portion of man's sphere of activity in the finite being, as Time and Space manifest the creative and motivative force." (1554-3)

In his book, *Vibrations*, Everett Irion notes that while time and space are forces outside of us, patience is strictly an internal activity. It should be added that patience is highly individual and reveals the spirit in which each of us lives and has lived throughout time. In a sense, then, time and space are witnesses to our activities.

Since patience is a lesson we must learn, it is the means through which we will come to fully understand our purpose—and who we really are—in time and space. These three principles are interrelated. Irion, however, states that they have to be comprehended individually. He proposes definitions for each, which are paraphrased here: *Time is the measure of our understanding of ideas; space is a measure of our understanding of the relationships among manifested ideas; and patience is a measure of our understanding of the purpose of manifested ideas.* These definitions help clarify the interface among the aspects of consciousness.

Together, they allow us to discern the purpose of our experiences, and to learn again that we are an integral portion of all creation, including those dimensions hidden from our senses.

Although it may not appear to be the case to our human senses, the physical world is a shadow of the spiritual world, according to the readings. The spiritual realm is the true reality, then, and the physical is an effect, a projection. We may feel that there is more to existence than meets the eye, as it were, which is the reason Cayce stated:

> " . . . as one finds self as a shadow, or as a representative of that indicated in the eternal—one may ask, what is the source of this association or connection?
>
> It is time, space and patience that bridges that distance. These are man's concept of the spirit of God manifesting to the three-dimensional consciousness." 2771-1

These dimensions are all that we manage to consciously grasp of God's presence and eternal dominion. The mundane mind is at a loss to comprehend fully its connection to the dominion. Left on its own, it never will; but fortunately it is not left entirely to its own devices. This is where sleep and dreaming come in.

The World of Dreams

Sleep and dreams are necessary, not only for the body, but also for the soul. Every night as you sleep, your soul leaves your body, thus it gets a rest from all the mundane clutter that has bombarded it during your waking hours. And while it is taking leave of your senses, the soul is taking stock and gathering material from that record you have written upon time and space throughout the eons.

As reading 5754-1 defines it: "sleep is a shadow of, that intermission in earth's experiences of, that state called death; for the physical consciousness becomes unaware . . . " except for the influences of subconscious forces. In normal sleep, the senses are on guard, with the auditory forces becoming more acute. Physical perception is shut down, but "the auditory sense is sub-divided, and there is the act of hearing by feeling, the act of hearing by the sense of smell, the act of hearing by *all* the senses that are independent of the brain centers themselves, but are rather of the lymph centers . . . " while the brain sleeps. This shift in bodily forces allows us to be more receptive to the impressions of the sixth sense:

> Of what, then, does this sixth sense partake, that has to do so much with the entity's activities by those actions that may be brought about by that passing within the sense *range* of an entity when in repose, that may be called—in their various considerations or phases—experiences of *something* within that entity, as a dream—that may be either in toto to that which is to happen, is happening, or may be only presented in some form that is emblematical— to the body or those that would interpret such.
>
> These, then—or this, then—the sixth sense, as it may be termed for consideration here, partakes of the *accompanying* entity that is ever on guard before the throne of the Creator itself, and is that that may be trained or submerged, or left to its *own* initiative until it makes either war *with* the self in some manner of expression—which must show itself in a material world as in dis-ease, or disease, or temper, or that we call the blues, or the grouches, or any form that may receive either in the waking state or in the sleep state, that has *enabled* the brain in its activity to

become so changed or altered as to respond much in the manner as does a string tuned that vibrates to certain sound in the manner in which it is strung or played upon.

Then we find, this sense that governs such is that as may be known as the other self of the entity, or individual. Hence we find there must be some definite line that may be taken by that other self, and much that then has been accorded—or recorded—as to that which may produce certain given effects in the minds or bodies (not the minds, to be sure, for its active forces are upon that outside of that in which the mind, as ordinarily known, or the brain centers themselves, functions), but—as may be seen by all such experimentation, these may be produced—the same effect—upon the same individual, but they do not produce the same effect upon a different individual in the same environment or under the same circumstance. Then, this should lead one to know, to understand, that there is a *definite* connection between that we have chosen to term the sixth sense, or acting through the auditory forces of the body-physical, and the other self within self.

In purely physical, we find in sleep the body is *relaxed*—and there is little or no tautness within same, and those activities that function through the organs that are under the supervision of the subconscious or unconscious self, through the involuntary activities of an organism that has been set in motion by that impulse it has received from its first germ cell force, and its activity by the union *of* those forces that have been impelled or acted upon by that it has fed upon in all its efforts and activities that come, then it may be seen that these may be shown by due consideration—that the same body fed upon *meats*, and for a period—then the same body fed upon only herbs and fruits—would *not* have the same character or activity of the other self in its relationship to that as would be experienced by the other self in its activity through that called the dream self. 5754-1

This commentary receives further clarification in follow-up reading 5754-2, in which Cayce explained that the sixth sense is an active force in the sleeping body. The question is then posed as to what relation this sense has with the mundane five senses. The sixth sense is the activating force of the "other self." What exactly is this other self? The answer is given in this profound statement: "That which has been builded by the entity or body, or soul, through its experiences as a whole in the material and cosmic world . . . or is as a faculty of the soul-body itself." Thus the functions of the mundane senses contribute to the experiences of the soul, and these experiences are aspects of the other self.

For the sake of simplicity, we might think of this other self as a projection of our individual existence since the beginning of time. While the body sleeps, the other self communes with the soul as it "goes *out* into that realm of experience in the relationships of all experiences of that entity that may have been throughout the *eons* of time, or in correlating *with* that as it, that entity, *has* accepted as its criterion or standard of judgments, or justice, within its sphere of activity."

If, through the subconscious (the soul's consciousness), the other self is made aware, for instance, of some action on the part of the sleeping body that disagrees or conflicts "with that which has been builded by that other self, then *this* is the warring of conditions or emotions within an individual." As a result of these interactions, this reading adds, someone may go to sleep feeling sad, but wake up feeling elated. Another individual may go to bed feeling elated, but awaken depressed, lonely, without a sense of hope, and in low spirits.

It is through these spiritual dynamics that we meet ourselves. We are revisited by what we have created. In the modern vernacular, what goes around comes around: "The experiences of the soul are meeting that which it has merited, for the clarification for the associations of itself with that whatever has been set as its ideal." As used here, *ideal* refers to any standard, whether advisable or unwise. Today we are the sum of all that we have been in the past—factored, perhaps, by the spiritual gains and losses we have merited. These intricate relationships help explain why good things may come to "bad" people, and vice versa. Just because you are a paragon of spirituality in this life doesn't necessarily mean that you are home free.

Language of Dreams

From these psychic revelations, we see that while sleep gives the body a chance to rest, it also serves a bigger purpose by allowing the soul an opportunity to take stock. The results are usually returned to us as dreams. Your dreams are feedback from the soul relative to your physical, mental, and spiritual states during your waking hours, and thus a source of guidance. The readings recommend that people record their dreams and study them. If you have difficulty recalling your dreams, simply give yourself a gentle suggestion several times as you lie in bed at night that you will remember them. It is also understandable why Cayce would state that dream recall is very important and that people who do not remember their dreams are negligent.

The readings point out that nothing important happens in your life that you do not dream about first. By recording and studying your dreams, you begin to un-

derstand what they are trying to tell you; and they often
have a lot to say. The fact that you are willing to become
receptive to these nightly status reports works—especially if you try to follow their guidance—to resolve the
"warring" within, a condition which would tremendously improve the quality of your sleep and dreams.

Cayce remarked in reading 5754-3 that we seek physical consciousness for our own diversion, but "In the sleep
[the soul] seeks the *real* diversion, or the *real* activity of
self." It is this schism that is the predicate for dreaming,
which we are assured is a natural activity "to make for
man a way for an understanding!" Understanding, however, does not come easily to the conscious mind when
nocturnal messages cross the gap between it and the subconscious. The primary difficulty in comprehending
many dreams, in fact, arises from the cause that makes
them necessary in the first place—the separate diversions
of the physical and the spiritual. They speak different
languages. On the physical side, understanding requires
linear, connected particulars of finite ideas. The soul mind
is oriented to the infinite and understands the principles
related to ultimate purpose beyond the reach of mundane awareness.

Thus, communicating meanings as allied with purpose makes transliteration difficult for the soul mind. It
has to translate its understanding through mundane images familiar to the conscious mind, but the images may
not always be sufficient to relay the meaning clearly. The
images, however, may be obscure for a number of reasons. They may not seem to present a logical sense or
context, or the dreamer may not remember all the details
presented. This is the reason recording your dreams is a
good idea. On occasion you will find that the same elements—if not the exact images—appear again and again
in different settings. And a dream may bear on more than
one aspect of your being, as reading 39-3 indicates when

it says that dreams are "the emanations from the conscious, subconscious, or superconscious, or the combination and correlation of each . . . "

Interpreting Your Dreams

If you have difficulty interpreting the import of a dream, ask what the dream means as you are going to sleep on the following evening; and continue asking nightly until you receive clarification through a subsequent dream or through an intuitive flash of understanding. By recording and studying your dreams, you will work out your personal symbolic references. While there are universal meanings behind certain images, these may or may not apply in individual cases. A bird may represent one thing to you and convey a different meaning to another person. All dreams are not symbolic, of course, and many are as straightforward as possible. Yet, even then a dream may seem peculiar or unsettling.

In *Why Do We Dream?* Everett Irion details the recurring dream of a young man who was chased night after night by a wild man. The pursuer sometimes held a gun and at other times a club, rock, or some other weapon. Just before his attacker caught up with him, the young man always snapped awake in terror. Irion advised the man to confront the attacker, which he could do by instilling the idea of facing him while going to sleep. During the dream in which he accomplished this, the pursuer was carrying a gun; but once the dreamer stopped fleeing, turned around, and opened his arms to the other, saying, "I know you're going to kill me, so go ahead and let's get it over with," the attacker instantly tossed the gun down, held out his hand, and exclaimed, "Thank God, you're going to talk to me. I have been chasing you for three years. Now we can talk."

No more is said about the result of this dream, but

presumably the message all along was the man had been ignoring the guidance offered, and this fact was dramatized in the dream until he got the message. And more likely, this dream reflected the warring within caused by his avoidance in dealing with matters vital to himself. As Irion comments: "It is evident that a part of the unconscious wanted his attention, but he . . . had to face this opposing facet of himself before he could understand its purpose."

In another case, a woman experienced a repetitive dream in which she saw skeletons. Again and again the skeletons appeared, a rather bizarre image to say the least, and she was understandably disturbed by these images continually dominating her dreams. Finally she asked what the dream meant, as she was going to sleep. That same evening she dreamed of seeing a pitcher pouring milk into a glass, and then it became obvious that her subconscious was not trying to spook her, but simply to let her know that her system needed more calcium.

These two dreams were warnings, one related to the physical, the other perhaps to mental and spiritual considerations. It may be that most dreams are warnings of a kind, in that they bring to mind aspects of ourselves or of our lives that need attention. Cayce was asked to interpret a woman's dream in which she was paralyzed and falling apart, as pieces of her body fell off or exploded. Frantically she cried out for her mother. Because of her intense suffering, she wanted to die. From his psychic state, Cayce replied:

> In this there is presented, as is seen from the experiences of the body conscious and the mental consciousness of the entity, through the subconscious, those projections of physical conditions and mental positions or manifestations that bring to the body-conscious mind this condition. It is as the warning

that the mental attitude and the body-conscious mind must gain a different concept of conditions being presented, that the full consciousness of the entity may not feel that this condition of paralysis to the mental portion of the entity, or that such conditions in the mental development, is at the standstill, or must be broken; else, as is seen, there is the call to that consciousness to whom the body conscious and the mental consciousness of the individual turns for the instruction, see?

Then the lesson—rather that the mental forces of the entity are to expand, rather than to fight, as it were, or try to deny that which the inner consciousness has made a portion of the entity. 136-39

The condition referred to had already been discussed in the first reading this woman received; it was noted that while she was slow to anger she held a grudge once riled, and Cayce added that she was "one who keeps the forces of wrath dominant in self when aroused." (136-1) This trait had been cultivated in a previous lifetime, and it was still a part of her temperament. The struggle to resist her vindictive inclinations, however, was creating a paralyzing influence, as demonstrated in the dream. Thus, Cayce suggested that instead of fighting or denying the urge she should expand her understanding, which would allow her to grow beyond this latent tendency and break away from it. And without question, the wisdom in this advice has its precedent in "resist not evil." Struggle only entrenches an evil or habit more deeply. Ingalese was certainly echoing the view of Cayce's interpretation when he observed that "it is by enlightenment that any and all our emotions are controlled or eliminated from us."

It is useful to remember that the impetus of your dreams is to help and guide, remind and warn. The meanings they convey may reach into any facet of your life and activities. The guidance ranges from the practical to the spiritual and can offer insights into business dealings, investments, diets, personal relationships, and health, and also bring inspiration, reassurance, a sense of peace, past-life glimpses, expansion of consciousness, spiritual understanding, and a keener awareness of divine influences in your life. When dreams are troubling or unsettling, they are trying to get your attention by pointing out some conflict within you or your life. A disturbing dream should be analyzed carefully and all elements considered.

A man [2671] reported a strange, complicated dream. Standing in his yard, he felt something inside the cloth of his coat that turned out to be a black cocoon, which broke open as he was removing it. A small black spider crawled out and began growing rapidly as it ran away. The spider was speaking in English, but all the man understood was that the creature was muttering something about its mother. Later he saw the spider, as large as his fist, inside his house. It had made a web "all the way across the back inside the house and was comfortably watching me." (2671-5) He knocked it down and out of the house with a broom and thought he had killed it, but the spider began talking again. He stepped on it and assumed again he had killed the spider, but later saw that it had built another web, this one outside the house, and was running up toward the eaves of the house when the man threw his straw hat in front of it, cutting the web and causing the spider to fall to the ground, where the man chopped up the spider with a knife.

Cayce explained the dream represented conditions that were going on in the man's personal life. The spider was a warning that he should take a definite stand regarding his relations with others. The man, who was married, had developed a relationship with another woman; and in short, the issue was adultery. Although Cayce did not say it outright, he implied that the man was about to become trapped in a web of deceit involving the other woman, with the warning that he was risking everything he had built. The gist of the counsel was this admonishment: "Take the warning then. Prepare self. Meet the conditions as the man, not as the weakling—and remember those duties that the body owes first to those to whom the sacred vows were given, and to whom the entity and body owes its position in every sense . . . " (2671-5)

This dream is an example of why the readings generally recommend that the dream needs to be correlated with what is going on in a person's life, because there is usually a direct connection, especially when it comes to images that augur a warning of some kind. Dream sequences may also be telepathic, or they can lead the mundane mind to the solution to problems, such as Howe's dream of spears with holes in the tips, which gave him the answer to developing a more efficient sewing machine. Because dreams are highly personal, they are often meaningless to anyone but the dreamer. Seeing snakes, for instance, is curious if not downright creepy, particularly if you dream of one biting its own tail. What does it mean? In 1865, chemist August Kekulé knew exactly what this dream meant: The snake holding its tail led him to discover the structure of the six-carbon benzene molecule, which forms a ring. The dream and the chemist's discovery revolutionized organic chemistry.

People whose work relies on imagination, such as artists and inventors, appear to receive guidance at times from their dreams for their creations. Numerous writers have solved creative complexities while their conscious minds rested. Two critical scenes in *Dr. Jekyll and Mr. Hyde* came to Robert Louis Stevenson via dreams, which enabled him to complete the novel.

Dreams are precognitive in many instances and sometimes foretell events years in advance. They may even foretell tragedy. President Abraham Lincoln dreamed of seeing a corpse laid out in a room of the White House a few days before he was assassinated. All dreams about death, however, are not necessarily literal. They may be symbolic, perhaps indicating an aspect of the dreamer that will end, or suggesting a pending change of some kind.

It is not unusual to dream of somebody who is dead, and in many cases these are telepathic contacts with the person's spirit. The contact may be meant only as reassurance that, though no longer in a body, the deceased is fine. At times the contact may be to offer information about the location of an item the deceased had stashed away. The spirits of the departed are also known to offer advice or opinions on any number of matters. Such counsel should be considered, of course, but not given undue credence in every case, simply because it comes from someone who is no longer living. As the readings point out, just because somebody is dead doesn't make the person any smarter than when he or she was living.

Telepathic dream communications with living persons are also common. As psychiatrist Carl Jung postulated, and the readings verify, all subconscious minds are constantly in touch. Irion cites an astonishing case of what apparently involved telepathy. In Pakistan an infant died and according to custom was buried the same day before sundown. (In Moslem countries, embalming is considered a desecration.) On three consecutive nights, the mother dreamed that her infant daughter was still alive. Each time, she woke her husband, who dismissed the dream without question. On the third night, however, she was adamant in demanding that the casket be unearthed and the body examined. A few neighbors helped them dig up the casket. When they opened it, the baby was busily sucking her thumb.

Dream Symbols

A great deal has been written regarding the appearance of symbols in dreams. The use of visual symbols makes sense if you consider that a visual image delivers a stronger impression than words. A tableau will remain in the mind long after words have faded from memory. Despite all the analytical reasoning about universal themes and archetypes imbedded in our psyches, the clearest way to think of symbols is as mental shorthand— keeping in mind that anything in a dream may mean more than might be apparent.

If the readings are correct in stating that physical reality is a shadow of the spiritual, then everything in this objective world has a larger meaning beyond that recognized by our mundane senses. The purpose of a dream is to communicate an awareness to the dreamer that the conscious mind is able to grasp; and for this reason the images transmitted are as literal as the subconscious mind can conjure to get the message across. Consider the following dream, which was presented to Edgar Cayce, and see if you can guess what it is trying to tell the dreamer:

A headless man in uniform of a sailor was walking in an erect manner with either a gun or a cane in his hand. 137-36

The young man mentioned this dream image at the end of a long reading that dealt primarily with business advice. The most striking point of the dream, of course, is the man with no head. On the surface the meaning appears obvious. But is the dreamer really being told that he has no head on his shoulders? What do you make of this image?

In his reply Cayce urged, "Do not lose the head too much in duty . . . " but to give attention to "the greater lessons as may be learned from the association of ideas as pertain to things more spiritual." The uniform represented the allegiance to duty, and perhaps the gun or cane highlighted his firm commitment. At any rate, Cayce's remark is quite practical considering that its roots are in the principle of balance, a quality which the readings always stressed. Just as attention to body and mind is necessary for one's well-being, so is attention to the spirit. Giving sufficient thought and consideration to each aspect of ourselves maintains harmony within. The import of this dream was literal with regard to the image; the man in uniform had lost his head. The missing head, however, was a symbol in the metaphorical sense. There was no risk of losing his physical head, but apparently he was at some risk of losing the perspective necessary for his continued spiritual growth.

It is always advisable to take dreams at face value and as literally as possible, and only look for symbolic meanings only when they remain unclear. A good example is a dream reported by a young man in reading 137-24: He was riding on a trolley car and lost his raincoat. "The trolley car ran over it," he told Cayce, who replied this was a health warning; he should use the coat—"keeping body dry, keeping feet dry"—to avoid illness. The meaning of the dream hardly required a clairvoyant interpretation. A bit of reflection would have made the man realize he was ignoring the purpose of the coat. A segment in another dream by the same man included a bottle of milk that was labeled "Undistilled milk." Since this was the type of milk he was consuming at the time, he was advised, "This should be changed to that of the Certified Milk . . . "

Most dreams appear to contain symbolic elements, and when they cannot be understood in literal terms, they must be analyzed carefully. The symbols should be considered in light of your understanding of or idea about them. Remember that, above all, dreams are personal reports, keeping in mind Cayce's advice in 900-8 that "all dreams are but the speech of the conditions in the mental, physical, or sub-conscious self." Thus, the symbols should be correlated with these facets to determine the dream's message. Irion observes, "From the intelligence within the soul, dreams contain the universals and eternals unknown to the conscious mind." It is primarily the eternal verities that concern the soul in time, space, and patience, where the soul seeks to apply these truths.

This same impetus was probably what generated the following episode by the young woman who dreamed that she was paralyzed. In an earlier reading, her fourth, she told the psychic about her dream of riding a horse and falling off the animal. Cayce told her that the horse and rider were "as the messenger that comes to each and every individual, and the falling off the rejection of the message . . . " (136-4) He also noted that she had not told all of the dream, which included a roadway with obstructions that made the horse shy, "causing rider to fall . . . [the obstructions representing] the conditions through which the mental forces must pass to reach the greater forces in an understanding manner."

Either the woman forgot to include the details about the obstruction or she had forgotten this part of her dream. Or maybe she left the details for Cayce's clairvoyant mind to address. Whatever caused her lapse, it serves as a good reminder why recording dreams, including even minor details, can lead to a clearer interpretation.

Recording Your Dreams

If you have never taken the time to record and analyze your dreams, you are in store for a fascinating journey into your own mind once you begin. Your willingness to be receptive to the messenger will be, well, soul-satisfying. The following are tips to help you get started recording your dreams. Just remember, the real key to understanding your dreams is patience:

- Keep a pen and writing pad or a tape recorder at your bedside. Whenever you wake with the memory of a dream, record it immediately. The longer you wait, the less you will recall about the dream. If you use a recorder, write down the dream in your log book when you get a chance. It will simplify comparing the dreams.
- Record even snippets or fragments that you recall. They may become more important when compared to elements in other dreams.
- Make special note of your dream state of mind, as well as emotional tones or attitudes, mannerisms, and reactions of others. Write down all the details related to the setting and atmosphere of the dream.
- Give special attention to repetitive dreams, which are repeated because you are not getting the message entirely.
- If an episode is undecipherable to you, ask for a rerun with clarification as you are dozing off.
- Spend at least a few minutes every day reviewing your dreams, looking for similar motifs or images and noting your impressions in the dream log.
- Examine your dream in relation to what is presently occurring in your daily life. If no connection is evident, then take a guess, noting it in your dream log.
- Remember, as you lie in bed waiting for sleep, to think several times: "I will remember my dreams when I wake up." And also remind yourself to pay close attention while a dream sequence is unfolding.

Lucid Dreaming

Dreaming while the conscious mind actively observes probably began with the advent of dreaming. It was mentioned by St. Augustine in the fifth century and is referred to in the Tibetan Book of the Dead. The term *lucid dreaming* was coined by Frederik Willems Van Eeden more than 100 years ago. During the last fifty years, several books on lucid dreaming have been published.

This kind of dreaming also occurs during the REM stage of sleep. You might think that we would be conscious of dreaming at least most of the time considering that the brain-wave activity during REM matches that of a fully alert brain. That we are normally unaware we are dreaming may trace to Cayce's explanation that dreaming is a function of the soul mind, not merely a brain activity. Yet it seems logical to assume that the brain has to be in a waking mode electrically, whether conscious or not, in order to remember a dream.

Possibly most people have experienced an occasional flash of lucidity when dreaming. Being a conscious observer of events as they unfold has its advantage in that the dream may appear even more vivid and easier to recall in detail. Anyone can learn to activate the conscious mind while dreaming, according to advocates of the phenomenon. But acting as a conscious witness to a dream is one thing, while consciously participating and controlling events is another. There are benefits to be gained, such as using lucid dreaming therapeutically to quell unconscious fears or in dealing with nightmares.

Intruding upon your dreams, however, may not be advisable. The idea that dreaming is an activity of the soul mind seems to preclude the wisdom of consciously barging in and redirecting the information or guidance provided. This appears almost as fruitless as not remembering your dreams at all. In reading 900-59 Cayce stated, "The conscious mind rarely gains the entrance to truth in the subconscious, save in rest, sleep, or when such consciousnesses are subjugated through the act of the individual . . . "

This implied caveat is worth observing for the fact that, if Cayce was correct about the cause of dreams, we should be willing to listen to what our souls have to say without interrupting or manipulating their messages, which can only happen when the conscious mind is sub-jugated. After all, we are here for a purpose. The soul understands and tries to communicate its truth to its physical component. And this truth issues through the subconscious to awaken the consciousness to purpose. This purpose is, in a word, spiritual.

KEEPING YOUR BALANCE

The one quality too many of us probably lack in our lives is balance—balance among body, mind, and soul. Attending to each according to its needs doesn't come naturally; the process requires dedication and persistence. But more often than not, our lives get caught up in a vortex of habit and routine, of unchanging patterns, that sweep us along through circumstances we choose either by commission or omission. Thus we become victims of our own imbalanced activities by not keeping our house in order. Imbalance does not come about through the pitch and toss of chance, but by our own carelessness or negligence.

For example, an athlete may concentrate exclusively on physical ability and competitive skills to the detriment of mental and spiritual attributes. On the other hand, a minister, priest, or rabbi may become so absorbed in spiritual pursuits that body and mind are ignored. A scholar or scientist may become fixated on intellectual issues and research while the body and spirit suffer from neglect. In each case, imbalance is present—and imbalance is the stuff insomnia is made of, not to mention even more dire conditions that plague humankind. Just as our bodies need a balanced diet, our minds and spirits need those influences that enliven their forces and contribute to their well-being.

It might be questioned that since your mind is always active in some fashion during your waking hours how it can be ignored. The use of the mind is not the issue, but *how* it is used. Mind is the builder, and it never sleeps. The question should be: What kind of thoughts have you allowed your mind to feed upon, because that is what it will build; those thoughts inevitably will return to curse or damn, bless or heal you. It should be kept in mind that the law of karma is not about retribution, but justice. Karma works in conjunction with the law of balance.

Ingalese made this point explicitly when he wrote, "It is through equilibrium that the great law of justice brings back to man precisely what he sends forth, and this is why he often finds in his everyday life that he must readjust himself. 'Be not deceived; God (the law) is not mocked; for whatsoever a man soweth that shall he also reap.'" Ingalese's views are textbook Cayce and are echoed throughout the readings, as in 3684-1: "For the manner in which ye treat thy neighbor is the manner in which ye are treating thy Maker. And be not deceived, God is not mocked . . . "

Sooner or later we come to the realization that a balanced life is the only existence that is constructive and meaningful. A middle-aged banker received reading 3352-1. He was suffering from disturbances of the heart, liver, lungs, and kidneys caused by a prolapse of his colon, which had developed from his neglecting to maintain regular eliminations, according to Cayce. Although he was seeking physical advice from Cayce for his condition, he was also treated to a lesson in the philosophy of living:

We find that these [conditions] arose as a result of what might be called occupational disturbances; not enough in the sun, not enough of hard work. Plenty of brain work, but the body is supposed to coordinate the spiritual, mental and physical. He who does not give recreation a place in his life, and the proper tone to each phase—well, he just fools self and will some day—as in this body in the present—be paying the price. There must be a certain amount of recreation. There must be certain amounts of rest. These are physical, mental and spiritual necessities. Didn't God make man to sleep at least a third of his life? Then consider! This is what the Master meant when He said, "Consider the lilies of the field, how they grow." Do they grow all the while, bloom all the while, or look mighty messy and dirty at times? It is well for people, individuals, as this entity, to get their hands dirty in the dirt at times, and not be the white-collared man all the while! These are natural sources. From whence was man made? Don't be afraid to get a little dirt on you once in a while. You know you must eat a certain amount of dirt, else you'll never get well balanced. For this is that from which all conditions arise. For of dust man is made, and to dust he returns. Because he doesn't look dirty once in a while is no sign he isn't dirty in mind, if not in body, if not in spirit. For these are one, ever one . . .

But take time to add something to your mind mentally and spiritually. And take time to play a while with others. There are children growing. Have you added anything constructive to any child's life? You'll not be in heaven if you're not leaning on the arm of someone you have helped. You have little hope of getting there unless you do help someone else.

Do that and live a normal life, and you'll live a heap longer. Be worth a heap more than the position you occupy. For it is not what you do but what you really are that counts. This shines through—what you really are—much more than what you say. 3352-1

From Cayce's comments, a portrait forms of a man who apparently was one-dimensional, as it were, in his approach to life. His eliminations were not the only thing he was negligent about. As is often the case, a problem in one area of our lives is indicative of problems in other areas. In the case of this banker, he had lost touch with the balance between recreation and rest. But was he all that different from many of us today who are locked into routines that are less than balanced? Like the man who dreamed of the headless sailor, many people have become drudges to a misguided idea of a "work ethic" and have lost their sense of fun, of play, of taking the time to enjoy simple pleasures. The failure to keep one's balance is practically a sign of the times.

Those things with which we are involved and preoccupied register within our psyches as our ideals. And indeed they are the standards we live by. The readings point out that in their sphere of awareness body, mind, and soul are one, thus the ideal must be one. As a standard, an ideal keeps you directed, like a beacon that prevents you from going adrift. The beacon is also a reflection of purpose. Consider the full implication of the following from reading 622-6: "The spiritual is the life, the mental is the builder, the material is the result of that builded through the purposes held by the individual entity."

We are also reminded in 3003-1 to consider each lifetime in the earth as an opportunity, because we each enter with a mission. Each of us is "as a corpuscle in the body of God . . . free-willed—and thus a co-creator with God." (3003-1) This life is to be lived purposefully, which is the reason for setting ideals. In turn, ideals help fulfill the mission. It is also through working with our ideals that we come to understand ourselves and others better; and through this understanding we become aware of our cocreative relationship with God.

Working with Your Ideals

When the Cayce readings speak of an ideal, they are not referring to some fanciful notion of unreachable accomplishment. On this point, the information is very practical. An ideal is a standard or pattern you use as a guide. It may help to think of it as a reference model in conducting your activities. Cayce defined an ideal as a "perfect standard." Establishing your spiritual ideal is the most important experience you can have in life, he asserted, and asked in 357-1, "Who and what is thy pattern?" There are also physical and mental ideals to be reckoned as well.

Psychologist Henry Reed, discussing ideals in *Edgar Cayce on Mysteries of the Mind*, mentions that our beliefs, conceptions, and expectations determine our experiences, that mental patterns create our reality. He then provides this insightful distinction between how ideas and ideals work: "It will make a difference whether or not ideals, and not just ideas, are among those patterns. A life centered on ideals will continue to grow fruitfully. A life centered on ideas alone, however, will run dry, because ideas can easily be satisfied." Reed contends that ideals never reach "perfect fulfillment." This may well be true in light of Cayce's statement that "You don't go to heaven, you grow to heaven." Working with ideals is not only relevant to that growth, but is necessary in order to stay on the spiritual path.

In addition, we are counseled to do what we know to do here and now. What you do now reaches through time and is added to the ongoing record of what and who you are in the next earthly life. We are constantly defining ourselves. It is comforting to know, as the readings assure us, that just trying to do the right thing is often taken as righteousness. Establishing ideals and making the effort to live by our understanding of them is the first step. This does not mean once you set down your physical, mental, and spiritual ideals that they will remain forever the same. Nor do you have to overload yourself with formidable challenges. Working with your ideals—and your dreams—is a gesture of cooperation to your soul mind, an action which will open your consciousness to its truth. Your intent, in time, will make all the difference. Ideals are a means of keeping your intent engaged in your development. The process is what counts most.

The process is simple. Take a sheet of paper and separate it into three columns. In each column from left to right, print the headings: *Physical, Mental, Spiritual*. You may want to add a date to this sheet. Then take a moment and reflect on a physical ideal you would like to work toward. Be specific—generalizations don't count. For instance, if you are not in the habit of drinking enough water daily, perhaps you will write: *Drink six glasses of water everyday*. You may decide to reduce your red meat intake and replace it with more vegetables. You may decide to walk everyday. Under *Mental,* list things you will do to enhance your mental capacity. Perhaps you have always wanted to learn a foreign language, study philosophy, or explore astrology. Then under *Spiritual,* write down ideals relative to the topic. Maybe you will decide to read the Bible every day, or the Koran, or the Talmud, or inspirational literature. You may want to make it a habit to pray daily.

Keep the list relatively short, no more than three to five items in each column. Spend a few minutes going over each ideal, and make any additions or changes that occur to you. You may also want to add when and where you will practice these ideals relative to time and situations. For instance, if you list regular exercise, you should indicate the time of day you will perform them; or if you have decided to be kinder toward others, you might list people you feel you have been unkind toward. Study the list carefully, and see yourself doing what you have written. For now, these are your ideals, the things you will apply. Commit them to memory.

Fold the list and place it in an envelope, seal the envelope and date it. Put the envelope away. Continue daily to apply the ideals in the three areas you indicated. If you miss a day, simply assure yourself that you will do better tomorrow—and from then on; don't make excuses for not exercising or failing to be kind to someone, etc. After four to six months, sit down again and repeat the process as if you are beginning for the first time, listing your ideals under the three columns. Study these a moment, then retrieve your first list and compare it with your new list. Make any changes or additions to the new list you feel are appropriate, incorporating both lists and writing down the results as your new set of ideals. Continue doing this for over a period of time, and you will discover that the three separate columns of ideals become more and more unified as one expression of your individuality, your purpose. Before you decide on your specific ideals, however, let's look at the three facets that combine to make you the person you are.

The Physical Body

Few things are taken for granted as habitually as the human body—until it rebels with pain, illness, or disease, then it demands our attention. Despite the stresses and abuses a body may be forced to undergo, it remains highly adaptable and resilient in adjusting to changes of activities and environment. The human body is an evolutionary marvel that lives and survives in every climate on earth from the blazing heat of equatorial regions to the frigid wastelands of the poles. It can subsist on an extremely limited variety of food.

The anatomical and muscular structure of the body gives it exceptional mobility to perform numerous movements. And while there are creatures that surpass us in a specific ability—such as the eagle with its visual acuity— none excels *Homo sapiens* in sheer versatility of physical accomplishments. The human body is nature's ideal creature.

And isn't this the way you see your body, as flesh and blood, organs and bones? Generally, this is also the way you think of it; that is, as a palpable entity, albeit a complex organism with numerous intricate and unified parts and with the most highly evolved brain on earth. You think of your body as who you are, and it *is* you, physically. It is your house while you live in the earth, and you are responsible for it as both inhabitant and custodian. Whatever the state of your body today, it is the result of how you have treated it not only in this life but also in your past lives. Your body is made in the image of your collective physical ideals through time and space.

But how is this possible? The body dies, so even if a soul returns, how can its body next time be like the previous body? This question is similar to the one Nicodemus asked Jesus concerning rebirth of a person. We have to remember that the material body is a manifestation of the soul. The activities of each earthly life registers in the soul body. It is a vibrational imprint or reference the soul brings back to the next human life, with some modifications that take place between lifetimes. And while you may think of your physical body as more or less a solid form, there is more to it than meets the eye. Your physique is an electromagnetic energy field composed of myriad unseen atoms. Consider Ouspensky's remark about subatomic particles:

> Electrons . . . are not material particles in the usual meaning of the word. They are better defined as moments of manifestation, moments or elements of force . . . It is possible to think that the difference between matter and force consists simply in different combinations of positive and negative electrons. In one combination they produce on us the impression of matter, in another combination, the impression of force . . . Matter and force are one and the same thing, or, rather, different manifestations of one and the same thing.

In a similar way, soul and body are a manifestation of the same thing. Each earthly life is a moment of manifestation for the soul. Together, body and soul assume a sacred relationship: spirit manifesting in matter. The readings contain numerous references to the body as the temple of God and as analogous to the Godhead of the trinity. In reading 1299-1, Cayce also observed, "the Father hath promised and has given us a body, that is a temple of the living soul . . . " Because we became enmeshed in the material plane, the development of the body, and its evolution, serve as a means for the soul to develop, to grow in grace, and return to its origin. To accomplish this, the soul is challenged to spiritualize its physical embodiment. The body, however, is involved in its own urges—with its self. Cayce often defined sin as self, as expressed in selfishness, self-aggrandizement, etc. The complication is that this expression of self operates in opposition to, and separates the soul from, full integration with the oneness of all creation and direct companionship with God, which it had in the beginning. The soul's relationship to its body is not unlike the Creator's relationship to the soul: God wants oneness of spirit with the soul, and the soul wants oneness of spirit with the body.

There is nothing inherently sinful or evil, however, about the body or its natural urges. Despite opinions to the contrary, the desires of the body are not to be repressed or ignored at all. In reading 3234-1, Cayce states that all desires have a place in human experience, but these desires are to be used, not abused: "All things are holy unto the Lord, that He has given to man as appetites or physical desires, yet these are to be used to the glory of God and not in that direction of selfishness alone."

This is reason enough to respect your body and its functions, giving them the care and consideration they require. Taking time for the body and its maintenance is not vanity; it's attending to the temple. Keep these points in mind as you select your physical ideals—as well as Cayce's suggestion in 294-7 to, "Keep the physical fit that the soul may manifest the longer." The longer the soul is in the earth, the more it can accomplish spiritually in its development.

The Mental Body

During the question-and-answer session of reading 1472-2, Cayce was asked whether a body loses all feeling at death, and, if not, how can it feel. He remarked that this depended on how unconsciousness is produced, or even on the way consciousness has been trained. He apparently was saying that there are two factors involved: the manner in which we die and our convictions about what happens after death. The readings refer to death as passing through "God's other door," and assure us that mundane consciousness may continue for a time after we pass through the door, which is what makes it possible for the dead to remember their feelings.

The soul's memories, and its attachment to them, are what motivate the soul to contact the living—"to make those impressions upon the consciousness of sensitives or the like. As to how long—many an individual has remained in that called death for . . . *years* without realizing it was dead!" In time the consciousness, which may remain with the soul after death, fades. When the moment of manifestation ends, the account of the soul's activities in the body remains as a record written in time and space.

The same questioner wanted to know, "If cremated, would the body feel it?" Cayce replied with the following enlightening comments:

> What body?
>
> The physical body is not the consciousness. The consciousness of the physical body is a separate thing. There is the mental body, the physical body, the spiritual body.
>
> As has so oft been given, what is the builder? *Mind!* Can you burn or cremate a mind? Can you destroy the physical body? Yes, easily.
>
> To be absent (what is absent?) from the body is to be present with the Lord, or the universal consciousness, or the ideal. Absent from what? What absent? Physical consciousness, yes.
>
> As to how long it requires to lose physical consciousness depends upon how great are the *appetites* and desires of a physical body! 172-2

These statements deal with two important ideas as to the nature of mind. It is with the mind, not simply the brain alone, that we recognize the sensations called feelings; and the mind does not die with the brain. Since it survives death, the mind can retain memories of its life as a personality as well as its emotions. Just how long these conscious memories linger is determined by how deeply attached we are to our physical sensations.

The mind does not require a body in order to function. In the body, the conscious mind is a finite expression of the soul's mind, which in turn is an individualized expression of the superconscious, the mind of God. The readings say that each individual is like a corpuscle in the mind of God. This analogy gives you good reason to think long and hard about what kinds of thoughts you habitually entertain. These thoughts, held long enough in the mind, become your ideals for good or bad. Fortunately, you have the ability to monitor your thoughts and use your will in determining which to maintain as ideals and which to replace.

Mind and will are the means that allow the soul to reckon and choose. Will is like a navigational system. Reed observes that the mind directs and shapes energy as patterns, but makes no qualitative distinction among them, because choice is not the mind's responsibility. "It is the job of the will," he explains. "We have choices about which mental patterns will shape the flow of energy in our lives."

The power of the will should not be taken lightly or expressed casually. Ingalese contends there are two important rules with regard to will. Together they offer a sensible reference: Neither speak nor act until you give thought with your subjective (soul) mind. The constructive use of will demands self-control in directing your energies with positive purposes. The conscious mind, allied as it is with the ego, is often given to less than constructive patterns. The subconscious, however, reflects divine energies that are not entirely hostage to selfish urges, because it is aware of its origin.

Ouspensky argues that, unless a person attains inner unity, he or she has no real "I" or will: "The concept of 'will' in relation to [a person] who has not attained inner unity is entirely artificial." Without unity, he explains, the "I" continually changes like a kaleidoscope, since our actions are driven by involuntary motives, which means "The whole life is composed of small things which we continually obey and serve." This is the same as saying that acting cued by reacting is not a true application of will, because the response isn't chosen; it is more akin to an automatic reflex. This is further reason to choose mental ideals that lay stepping-stones toward inner unity.

The Spiritual Body

Soul and spirit are conventionally understood to mean the same thing. Strictly speaking, the two terms are not exactly synonymous, according to the readings, which reveal that spirit is the "activating force" (the divine spark), and soul is the individual entity, the individuality of that force endowed with mind and will. In the physical world, this divine spark may be either accessed or ignored. This depends on whether you cultivate spiritual ideals or take an indifferent posture to your essence, or perhaps even reject the idea that the soul exists at all.

To work with spiritual ideals is to draw the activative essence of your being to manifest in all your physical and mental activities. This, in turn, patterns your energies into a unity of purpose; and then you not only understand that you know yourself to be yourself, you also know you are one with God. In this oneness you realize your purpose.

The readings teach that the most important pursuit of

any individual is to determine the spiritual ideal. "Who
and what is thy pattern?" Cayce asked in one reading. He
then commented:

> Throughout the experience of man in the material
> world, at various seasons and periods, teachers or
> "would be" teachers have come; setting up certain
> forms or certain theories as to manners in which an
> individual shall control the appetites of the body or
> of the mind, so as to attain to some particular phase
> of development.
>
> There has also come a teacher who was bold
> enough to declare himself as the son of the living
> God. He set no rules of appetite. He set no rules of
> ethics, other than "As ye would that men should do
> to you, do ye even so to them," and to know "Inas-
> much as ye do it unto the least of these, thy brethren,
> ye do it unto thy Maker." He declared that the king-
> dom of heaven is within each individual entity's
> consciousness, to be attained, to be aware of—
> through meditating upon the fact that God is the
> Father of every soul. 357-13

Scholars generally depict Jesus as a reformer. Reform-
ing was not His purpose, but to remind us of our true
nature, which is divine. Yet, when He said the kingdom is
within, it was a radical idea to propose that God is acces-
sible within each of our sinful bodies. It is noteworthy
that Jesus forgave sins of the flesh without question, but
sins of the spirit were brought to mind. The readings
explain the difference this way: "Sins are of commission
and omission. Sins of commission were forgiven, while
sins of omission were called to mind—even by the Master." (281-2)

Sins of omission arise from the failure to do what you
know to do, and the failure to live in the proper spirit.

Sins are reckoned by our attitudes toward and judgments of others; and we are warned that the faults we condemn in others are the ones we already possess. But whether our sins lean toward action or inaction, they answer to the two great commandments: Love God and love one another. They are the ultimate ideal, and they are the same thing, because each of us is a corpuscle in the body of God. We only need to look behind the mask of personality to understand that each of us is an individual soul, yet one in spirit.

In working with spiritual ideals, set small goals. Avoid the idea it is only the grand gesture that counts. A woman who felt an intense desire to serve God asked during a reading (1877-2) what she could do in particular. She was advised that it is not by might or great deeds that we serve God, but "here a little, there a little, line upon line . . . *sowing* the fruits of the spirit, *leaving* the fruition of same to God!"

The readings also inform us that each soul enters the earth to meet its self, its own shortcomings. Or to put it another way: Each life is an opportunity to shape the moment of manifestation into a pattern that is more in the image of the Divine. Applying the fruits of the spirit— kindness, gentleness, patience, love, etc.—is one of the ways we direct our energies into this pattern. God is Love, Love is Law, Law is God, asserted Cayce in numerous readings. And because a spark of the Divine is our essence, we have the capacity to reflect that Love in our lives. It is the light of this spark that will lead us from our shortcomings, and eventually from the shadows of ignorance about who we really are.

In *Reflections on the Path*, psychologist Herbert Puryear offers the reminder that Jesus' commitment to His ideal serves as our example. He remarks, "The pattern is written in us; it need only be awakened by the ideal we set, our application of it in our daily lives and our reliance on the truth of His example."

Perhaps it should be added that relying on Jesus as your example transcends religious boundaries, just as Mahatma Gandhi realized and his own life demonstrates. Johannes Eckhart *(Meister Eckhart)*, the fourteenth-century Christian mystic, declared, "God is love, so loving that whatever he can love he must love, whether he will or not." Eckhart meant that spirit answers to spirit. It was in the spirit of love that Jesus lived, and thus became the pattern for us all. He is the Master for the reason that He is the first earthbound soul to regain perfect oneness with God. Having freed Himself from the pull of physical forces, He gained mastery over the elements.

When you write down your ideals, following the procedures explained earlier, include only those ideals under the three headings that you feel are right for you at this time. Remember, the quest is for balance, so don't overload one column with ideals that will distract from the time you need to apply the others. In a few months, you will make another list and incorporate the ideals. If you are uncertain about just which ideals to list under any of the categories, you might consider praying. Meditation isn't a bad idea either.

Meditate and Know

During the last century, meditation gained a following in America. The number of practitioners remains relatively small, but that this Eastern discipline has found a niche not only here but also in Europe is a sign that our outwardly directed mindset is beginning to venture inward. Yet, our cultural orientation does not take easily to being still and changing mental states. We have too much on our minds, too much to do—which is one of the reasons quality sleep is scarce. Besides, meditation seems unnatural and strange. Henry Reed observes that this practice may conjure images of strange postures, shaven heads, and colorful robes, as well as exotic chants and religious cults, but he contends it is more ordinary than its publicity suggests, and more important than most of us realize, adding that "Cayce stressed it above any other activity, except for the setting of ideals, and it has the support of a substantial body of scientific evidence."

In some quarters, meditation is taught as a means of relaxation and controlling certain bodily conditions such as high blood pressure. Transcendental Meditation™ is promoted as a technique for reducing stress in addition to developing your potential. It is estimated that more than five million people use this technique. Studies have found that meditators experience numerous benefits from the practice, including better health and more vitality, sharper thinking, and increased happiness.

The readings also contain numerous references to the benefits meditation provides. Cayce recommended it as a method for receiving guidance in decision making; first deciding consciously, then going into the meditative state and asking your question so that it can be answered yes or no. The answer will come from your subconscious. Meditation is a spiritual practice, especially in conjunction with setting ideals. The readings comment that prayer is when you talk to God, and meditation is when God talks to you. It is in meditation that you come to a clearer understanding of Spirit answering to spirit.

While it has practical applications and rewards, it is clear from the readings that meditation should not be entered into casually. It is one thing to sit and relax your mind, but quite another to shift into the meditative state. Preparation is required. The shift is like going through uncharted territory. You need to know why you are there and what the risks are.

When you meditate, the life force—referred to as kundalini in Eastern mysticism—rises through the body and flows through the seven spiritual centers, which are situated in the area of the seven endocrine glands as the soul's contact points with the body. By being still and shutting down conscious thought, you open the way for the force to move unimpeded and unadulterated by physical urges. When this happens, you are opening yourself to psychic and spiritual influences—and potentially to influences that aren't spiritual at all in the divine sense.

This is the reason the Edgar Cayce discourses give procedural guidance with the recommendations to meditate. From beginning to end of the meditative state, four steps are advised: a prayer of protection, the Lord's Prayer, an affirmation. When the centers are fully opened and receptive, they are vulnerable to undesirable vibration as well as to the life force. The prayer of protection is like posting a divine guard to deflect uninvited influences. The Lord's Prayer, according to the readings, opens the centers; each part of the prayer relates to a specific center. The affirmation is repeated a few times in the first minutes following the Lord's Prayer to keep the mind focused on the ideal. When the meditation period ends, the Twenty-third Psalm is used by some meditators to close the centers.

Following these instructions is the safest approach for the beginning meditator as well as anyone experienced at the discipline. The readings also include other preparations to facilitate the process, such as specific breathing and head-and-neck exercises. If you are interested in meditating, read *Meditation—Gateway to Light*, by Elsie Sechrist. (See the references section.)

Obviously, keeping your balance requires a trilateral perspective of your being as body, mind, and soul. If one is neglected or overindulged, the others suffer from neglect also. A reasonable, moderate approach in working with tenable ideals and taking a few minutes each day to pray and meditate will anchor your life to purpose. Then you will sleep like a baby. But if on occasion you don't, consider Cayce's advice in reading 2051-5 to an older man who had difficulty sleeping after four in the morning: "This should not be attempted to be controlled, but rather *used* advantageously. If ye are aroused, use the period of the first thirty minutes—at least—in direct meditation upon what thy Lord would have thee do that day. You'll soon learn to sleep more than the next hour!"

Balance is not built in a day, of course, but it comes with persistence. Persistence requires patience, so there is no need to force matters. As Cayce reminds us, just trying to do the right thing is often taken as righteousness. Even when you have reached a point where you are more in balance and quality rest comes naturally, there are also outer conditions and circumstances to evaluate. So while you are in the process of improving your equilibrium, there are other factors to take into account, which we will look at in the final chapter to follow.

9

THE SLEEP SCENE

Sleep is a function of the human body that does not always come naturally. When it doesn't, something obviously is wrong. Insomnia is a hydra-headed symptom rooted in numerous causes, which have become so prevalent that an industry, sleep medicine, has developed to treat the disorders. There are treatment centers in almost all the American states, as well as throughout European countries. (A list of sleep associations is included in the resources section.) These centers are helpful if you cannot get a handle on your insomnia, and especially if you have a serious medical condition that contributes either directly or indirectly to your sleeplessness. If you suffer from sleep apnea, narcolepsy, sleep walking, or any other unusual chronic disorder, you should see a doctor who specializes in sleep-related disturbances.

In the majority of cases, insomnia seems to be circumstantial—related to working hours, lifestyle, etc.—thus largely within the control and cure of the sufferer, as indicated in preceding chapters. These final pages deal with additional factors and information to take into account, including specific suggestions regarding immediate issues and strategies to follow for the long term to help the natural quality of your sleep. Some of this information, of course, may appear obvious to any thinking person and involve matters about which you are already aware but nevertheless give these matters thought.

Your Sleep Environment

Bedding—The first item to evaluate in your sleep quarters is your mattress, which should be firm. A firm mattress is also generally recommended for anyone with back problems, according to orthopedic experts. A unit that sags at all or contains lumpy areas means that you should buy a new mattress set. If you decide to buy a new mattress, be sure to look at all the features carefully, because all units are not alike. If you opt for a waterbed for the sake of change, select one with baffles, which prevent the mattress from undulating from the wave effect of the water; you don't want to feel as if you are being tossed around on a raft in the middle of the night. If you sleep with a partner, you will probably find that the roominess of a queen- or king-sized mattress is better for double occupancy.

Consider your pillow and make sure it provides both comfort and adequate support. Some people find that they prefer down-filled pillows over the foam type, because the feathery support conforms naturally to the shape of their heads. To determine if a pillow is suitable for you, stand with your shoulder against a wall, then place the pillow between your head and the wall; it should fill the space comfortably. Regardless of what position you are in when you go to sleep and when you wake up, you spend much of the night on your sides. Also give some thought to the sheets you sleep on. If they are made of synthetic material, experiment with other fabrics, such as cotton, to determine whether they feel more comfortable.

Noise—One of the biggest nuisances to sleep is noise, almost any kind of noise. People who live near airports often claim they have become accustomed to the roar of planes taking off and landing while they sleep. Studies, however, reveal contrary facts. People who sleep amid the kind of noise generated by jet planes do not get the quality of sleep they imagine, because the high decibel count affects the autonomic nervous system whether the sleeper is aware of it or not. You *can* become used to certain noises and sleep well, on the other hand, if the sound is constant and not excessively loud.

If you live in an area where loud noise is the norm, there are steps you can take. Heavy drapes will buffer many exterior sounds. Also, some people who find virtually any sounds especially unsettling have gone so far as to line the walls and ceiling of their bedrooms with soundproof materials, including installing thick carpet on the floor, with underlaid padding as well. Taking similar measures is particularly helpful if you work nights and must sleep during the day in a noisy environment. Some people find soft earplugs helpful. Others have found that constant low-level sounds such as the steady drone of a fan acts as a screen that makes outside sounds more tolerable. There are also machines that produce sounds that mask other extraneous noises. Playing soothing music also helps by providing a relaxing mood.

Light—Light is another sleep robber. You will want to keep your room as dark as possible. Even very dim light passes through your closed eyelids, so make sure that no extraneous light comes through the windows. Even small amounts of light can cause too much stimulation for you to relax completely. If you have blinds, add curtains or drapes over them. If you now have thin curtains, buy a set thick enough to block out light. Avoid using a night light in your bedroom. If you have an illuminated digital clock on your bedside table, you might want to turn its face away from you. Even better, set it on the floor out of sight.

Temperature—Temperature is another factor to evaluate. Many people prefer a cool room in the range of sixty-five degrees Fahrenheit (eighteen degrees Celsius). You may prefer either a slightly warmer or cooler room, depending on whether you prefer a cover of some kind. By experimenting with different settings, you will be able to determine your comfort zone. Temperatures higher than seventy-five degrees have been found to affect the quality of sleep with increased awakening and less time in the deep stages of sleep. When noise isn't a problem, some people also prefer fresh air and raise a window at bedtime, even leaving it slightly open during the winter months while they sleep. If you do not have air conditioning, you probably use a fan. If it is hot enough to justify aiming airflow at your body, avoid having the air blow directly into your face.

It's Bedtime

Of all the reminders your parents uttered when you were a child, chances are the one you disliked most was, "It's your bedtime." You probably reasoned that bedtime is when you go to bed, but if you were not ready to turn in yet, then it should not be time. The logic in your reasoning was, and still is, irrefutable but self-defeating. At any rate, the following points are also reminders about your bedtime:

- **Maintain a regular bedtime.** Remember, if you pursue the heaven of late hours on weekends, there will be hell to pay come Monday when you have to drag yourself from the bed after spending half the night awake because your circadian rhythm is out of whack. If you do stay up past your normal bedtime, say on Friday night, rise at about your regular hour Saturday morning and make up the deficit that night. By sleeping in, you will not feel sleepy at your usual time, thus you will begin a vicious cycle of losing and resetting your rhythm week after week.

• **Have a bedtime routine.** By more or less following the same nightly preparations before turning off the lights and settling into bed, you condition your body to the expectation of sleep. You may want to follow Cayce's advice to drink several ounces of milk with a teaspoonful of honey stirred into it. He also recommended to at least one person to sip a little salted lemon juice to aid in sleeping. Remember, citrus juices are alkaline-reacting in your body. In addition, if you have a snack, be sure to keep it light; avoid overloading your stomach.

• **Avoid conflicts and stimulating discussions prior to bedtime.** There is something about nightfall that either arouses many people's grave emotions or evokes their philosophic brooding about everything under the moon. And the later the hour, the more urgent they feel the need to have their say. But when you are approaching the time to call it a night, refrain from ventilating and ruminating on matters that will look different come the light of day. Instead, settle into a relaxed, pleasant mood. Try to imagine, until morning, that you do not have a care in the world. If on occasion you get stirred up, soaking in a warm tub will usually put you in a relaxed state of mind. Showers, however, are not suitable for this purpose.

• **Reading or watching television shortly before you turn in** receives mixed reviews from sleep researchers. Some believe it is not advisable to get the mind too revved

SEEKING INFORMATION ON

holistic health, spirituality, dreams, intuition or ancient civilizations?
Call 1-800-723-1112, visit our Web site, or mail in this postage-paid card for a FREE catalog of books and membership information.

Name: _____

Address: _____

City: _____

State/Province: _____

Postal/Zip Code: _____ Country: _____

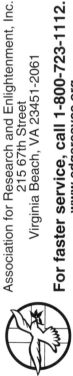

Association for Research and Enlightenment, Inc.
215 67th Street
Virginia Beach, VA 23451-2061

For faster service, call 1-800-723-1112.
www.edgarcayce.org

PBIN

up; others deem it is okay as long as you watch a boring show or read something light. A good rule might be not to get engrossed in anything that you have to stay up an extra hour to watch or read. Many researchers agree that the bed should be used only for sleep and making love, but they don't all agree about other activities, such as reading in bed.

Psychologist James Perl *(Sleep Right in Five Nights)* takes the position that if reading or watching TV helps, fine; but if it is stimulating to you, then it is best to do these in another room. He reasons that reading is preferable to tossing and turning and observes: "If reading always leads to sleep, over time sleep will become a conditioned response to reading. Eventually you will associate reading in bed with falling asleep, so that the stimulus of reading in bed helps elicit the sleep response." The same, he adds, is also true of watching TV or listening to music.

• **Shun strenuous exercise.** If you work out in the evening, finish at least three or four hours before bedtime. There are two mild exercises, however, mentioned in the Cayce readings that may help you relax and sleep better. The first is a stretching routine similar to that given earlier. When you are ready to go to bed, try this exercise, preferably with few clothes on and barefoot: Stand with your feet about shoulder-width apart, arms at your sides. Keeping your arms straight, but not rigid, slowly raise them in front of you. As they are coming up, begin rising gently on the balls of your feet, and stretch your arms, without straining, toward the ceiling for three to four seconds. Slowly lower your arms and heels to the starting position. Repeat ten times. If you have difficulty balancing on the balls of your feet in the beginning, lift your heels only slightly for several days until you become accustomed to the routine. This movement was recommended as a slimming exercise when repeated mornings and evenings. It also strengthens the internal muscles that support the organs.

The second routine, the head-and-neck exercise, can be performed just before turning out the light. Do these movements either standing or sitting, but make sure your back is comfortably straight. Relax your shoulders, then slowly, gently lower your head forward as if you are putting your chin on your chest without straining. Once your head is tilted as far as it will go, pause for a second, and then slowly return to the upright position. Repeat this movement three times with only a slight pause after each. Then tilt your head backward slowly, following the same procedure as before and holding for a second. Also repeat to the left and then to the right as if you were placing your ear against your shoulder. Once you have stretched in all four directions, rotate your head to the left in a full circle three times and then to the right. Imagine your head is attached to a string. Your movements should be relaxed and easy.

When performed daily, these two exercises are very relaxing. The stretching routines help tone muscles that may rarely get much use. The head-and-neck exercise is recommended in the readings as a preparation for meditation. Cayce also stated that it improves hearing and vision. Some persons reportedly have been able to do away with reading glasses after using this exercise mornings and evenings for several months. If done nightly at the same time just before you turn in, the exercises help remind the body that it is time to relax and sleep.

If you want to make certain you sleep well on a particular night, you may want to try Harold J. Reilly's recommendation and apply a cold pack to your abdomen, which he declared "will relieve insomnia when all else fails, and is excellent for the stimulation of the liver, kidneys, and other organs." He suggested that you may want to cover your bed with a rubber sheet or waterproof material up to twenty-four inches wide and sixty inches long placed crosswise on it. Use a towel or cloth that is long enough to wrap around your waist. Soak a thick cloth or towel thoroughly in water below sixty-five degrees. Loosely wring this out, then fold lengthwise to about a nine-inch width. You may place the cold towel on the larger one and wrap it around you after lying down; but it may be simpler to wrap the cold cloth around your waist and then cinch this with the longer towel before you lie down. The physiotherapist suggested, "Be certain it is tight and in contact with the skin at all points. If too long, it can overlap in front of the abdomen. Be sure the pack is airtight for proper reactions." It may be for the same reason that some experts suggest a cold shower is an excellent preparation for assuring sleep.

Other Reminders

If you are accustomed to taking an afternoon nap and have difficulty sleeping at night, isn't the solution obvious? Some people can nap and still sleep well at night, but others cannot eat their cake and have it, too. If you must take an afternoon nap, then shorten the time if you're not sleeping well at night. Researchers observe that naps tend to disrupt the sleep-wake rhythm, yet have also found that twenty percent of insomniacs have improved sleep at night if they nap during the day. James Perl observes, "These people seem to feel less anxious about going to bed at night if they know they have had a nap that day or can count on a nap the following day. This lowered anxiety level helps them relax at night and improves the quality of their sleep."

Avoid coffee and other caffeinated beverages in the evening. Do not use tobacco for at least two hours before bedtime. If you awaken during the night, do not smoke; nicotine stimulates your nervous system, and it will likely delay you from falling asleep again. Some people claim that coffee does not keep them awake. This may be true, but your sleep will be qualitatively better when no stimulants are in your system. Remember that caffeine comes in many forms, including chocolate and certain medications. Perl notes that insomniacs often rely on caffeine to fight fatigue after a night of poor sleep. "This caffeine consumption in turn can lead to another night of poor sleep, which then leads to more caffeine. The habit of using this drug to cope with insomnia can result in a continuing cycle of caffeine use and sleeplessness."

If you do not fall asleep within thirty minutes after climbing into bed, get up and involve yourself in a low-key activity such as writing letters. Perhaps the time might be used to work on those items listed under *Spiritual* in your ideals list. You might also want to take Cayce's advice to pray and meditate. Or if you insist on remaining in bed, you might want to have an audiotape handy that coaches you through relaxation exercises or guided imagery, such as "Getting a Good Night's Sleep," which provides a narrative of relaxation and presleep suggestions—with no subliminal messages. (See the resources section at the end of this book.)

Do not rely on alcohol for sleep, because it defeats your purpose. Peter Hauri points out in *No More Sleepless Nights* that "in nearly everyone, even if they've had only one or two drinks, drinking alcohol late in the evening produces troubled and fragmented sleep. The person does not sleep soundly, but wakes up many times throughout the night." Alcohol may help you get to sleep, yet you end up getting less sleep than if you had not consumed any.

As already discussed, your problem with sleep may be caused by any of a number of factors. If you are like most people, you have the remedy for solving your insomnia and getting the good night's sleep you deserve. All you need to do is make whatever adjustments are necessary in yourself, your circumstances, or your lifestyle. But considering that all causes are not equal, and some are not evident, how can you judge whether your insomnia is serious enough to warrant treatment by a professional? In his book, Peter Hauri provides the following guidelines for determining whether a sleep problem requires further help:

- You have suffered from insomnia for several months and it adversely affects the way you function during the day
- You have had an accident or near-accident at your home, place of work, or while driving
- Your job or personal relationships have been jeopardized by lack of sleep
- You believe or have been told that when asleep you have difficulty breathing or exhibit other signs of abnormal behavior such as bed-wetting or leg twitching
- You struggle to stay awake during the day
- Your mental acuity is diminished, and you experience spells of disorientation and forgetfulness

Hauri, director of the Mayo Clinic Insomnia Research and Treatment Program, states that any one these conditions is reason to see your doctor. If the doctor cannot help you, then ask for a referral to a sleep disorders center. "In any case," he emphasizes, "if your problem is serious and chronic and you can't handle it—whether it's that you can't get to sleep, can't stay asleep, or can't stay awake during the day—get help." Sleep centers have the diagnostic tools as well as the experience to help resolve your disorder.

Other Choices

One of the key recommendations contained in the Cayce readings is that we should take time to relax. Relaxation is an essential aspect in balancing our activities as well as our lives. Most of us know this, but how many of us stop to take the time? What we sometimes overlook is that sitting or lying around does not necessarily mean we are relaxed, because relaxation involves more than simply being idle. At times, assistance is needed just to relieve tensions that affect the nervous system in order to help restore the ability for normal rest throughout the body. When a woman asked how to ease her nervous condition, Cayce advised her in 3120-2 that relaxing at regular intervals was the best, and definitely better than depending on drugs. Extra amounts of B vitamins and particularly B-1 were recommended, but Cayce also repeated his suggestion for her to "Have a period when you forget everything—not necessarily to go to sleep to do so—but if you go to sleep during those periods, very well, but let the recuperation come from deep within self."

The case of another woman involved a diagnosis that is all too common in the readings. She wanted to know what caused her sleeplessness. This was brought on, Cayce informed her in reading 3386-2, by the incoordination between her cerebrospinal and sympathetic systems. The incoordination was causing a number of problems, including restless, disturbed digestion at times and headaches. This reading prescribed a regimen of internal cleansing, along with osteopathic corrections and massage as "a gentle relaxing treatment with specific attention given in the 3rd cervical, the 2nd, 3rd and 4th dorsal, 9th dorsal and through the lumbar area."

Similar advice was given to a man who wanted to know what could be done for his insomnia: "When these pressures are relieved in the cerebrospinal nervous system, the normal activity would be for a more normal rest." (5503-2) Physical stresses and tensions result in conditions that impair the body's flow of energy through the nerve forces and its ability to bounce back readily, which is why Cayce suggested to the man that he needed to create "an equilibrium from the extremities to the body" by using the Radio-Active Appliance, a special device that aids in restoring the balance of the subtle energies in the body.

Using this device as an aid to energy balance is mentioned in numerous readings. Ms. [911] was told, "This will bring sleep without any sedative from the outside, creating all necessary forces from within." (911-2) The woman wondered whether she should take hypnotics to help her relax and sleep, but Cayce warned her to stay away from artificial sleep inducers and assured her that the use of the Radio-Active Appliance would act as a natural hypnotic within her system. In reading 826-3, Cayce was explicit in stating that the device is helpful to anyone, "and especially those that tire or need an equalizing of the circulation; which is necessary for anyone that uses the brain a great deal—or that is unactive on the feet as much as is sufficient to keep the proper circulation."

The appliance is referred to in about a thousand readings, which include details of its construction. It is a kind of "battery" that enhances and balances the energies of the body. This unusual battery has to be "charged" in a special way. It has a measurable electrical current, but the current usually cannot be felt. When in use, two leads are plugged into the battery, then the other ends with special connections are attached to an ankle and to the wrist on the opposite side of the body. If the idea of the battery sounds peculiar to you, consider Cayce's comments in reading 1800-4, which explain the appliance provides the same benefits as sleep: "The whole organism of the human body made up of such electronic forces as is necessary for sufficient rest in that called sleep to recuperate the energies of the whole body. This application produces, then, that same effect in the system."

Whatever the illness or condition that manifests organically, it has its counterpart on an atomic level; and just as the body can be stimulated to heal itself by organic means, it can also be stimulated electronically toward the same healing.

The text of the following is presented in its entirety to give you an idea of what Edgar Cayce's psychic readings were like for those who sought his help. This reading was for a forty-three-year-old psychiatrist. Although she mentioned no specific ailment, note that in Cayce's diagnosis of her condition the clairvoyant delves into her physical condition on an atomic level. Illness reveals itself first in the body's electrical forces. This is also an excellent example how Cayce did not restrict his observations only to the physical:

> As to the physical conditions that we find existent, that which may be most helpful for the body would be in keeping or maintaining the nearer correct or normal affinity between the elements that make up the physical, the mental and the spiritual bodies. This would be more in accord with that which might be helpful. For, with this body more than most bodies, as we find, a conscious effort on the part of the body may make for almost whatever type of reaction physically that might be desired for the body.
>
> True, there are physical conditions that at times make for some disturbance; yet when the body stops itself to analyze same the body-mental is capable of knowing and experiencing not only the cause but

that which to the great measure may correct that physical condition.

A material body in a material world, to be sure, is subject to material laws; and a mental body that manifests through a perfectly balanced material body may see and experience and be conscious of the mental body from quite a different angle, or make quite a different approach to the physical aspects or experiences of bodies, as well as function in such a manner in relation to spiritual things as to use the attributes. Or, to become conscious in a material world it is necessary that some attribute of a normal body be made aware or conscious of that activity in its action, in its expression, in manifestation in material things.

Hence, as we find, from the physical angle or viewpoint, these conditions exist in this body, [444] we are speaking of, present in this room:

As to the *blood supply*, we find a body efficient in the proper division of the blood cells in numbers, both as to white and red blood supply. The division in the warriors within the white blood is near normally balanced, and that which acts rather as the plasm for recuperative forces in used tissue— whether related to the mental attributes or physical forces of the body.

The plasms of the activity of blood supply, as related to either the ohms or the urea or the elements in the hemoglobin, are well balanced; because mostly the body desires it so to be. For, the body may manifest itself that it may increase circulation where or when it desires to do so. This would be a very good experience for the body to show for itself those variations that may be made in pulsations in varied portions of the body. Not merely as a phenomenon or experimentation, but that—when there is the cause and the need—there may be the increased activity through the blood stream, which is evidenced or recognized in material things as being the life flow of a physical body. Be capable of doing this and applying same in the correct manner.

The *nervous system:* In the nerve plexus we find there have been occasions when the activities of the body-mental and body-physical have not always coordinating as to that which was or is to be the control in the body.

Hence we find there are ganglia about the cerebrospinal system that show impulsive reaction between sympathetic and cerebrospinal activity.

Don't consider nor get the idea that this is a physical derangement to harm, unless allowed to become excessive to such measures as to produce incoordination in impulses throughout the body.

Impulses receive their activity both from the soul's manifestation in a physical body and that the body-consciousness is aware of as impelling activity upon the physical organisms of the body.

Hence that great discussion (which has been interesting to this body) as to which is the most impelling in the influence of an active mind, environment or heredity; or, does blood tell or does the mental mind tell the most in that which may influence or be the most consistently active in the experience of an individual entity, body, mind or soul?

Then, in giving the physical attributes of this body here, let's treat them as *one,* but knowing they exist in the physical body as one; as also does the flexus of any muscular force in the body become impelled by that it is fed upon in its physical activity, as well as being acted upon that it may be aware of through any of the mental consciousness of the body—and thus become the more concerted in its activity as to that the body-mind, the mental-body, the soul-body, feeds upon and acts in itself as related to that it has become conscious or aware of.

In relation to this, it may be asked by the body: Through what channels does this activity occur, or this condition that is spoken of as being physically present in relation to the ganglia of the nervous system?

Through assimilation of influences from without, there is the activity upon various portions of the system to impel or create or give out that which not only makes for the sustaining of the activity but supplies the ohms, in the urea of the system, that which reproduces itself in its propagation in the physical body.

Hence, as the activities in this particular body have been along so many varied lines, so many activities as related to spiritual activity, mental associations, physical attributes being impelled or controlled by these, these have been so accentuated as to make for these physical conditions existent.

What supplies this ohm, what supplies the urea necessary for the constitution of the activities in the physical system? This is done through the secretions of glands as related to the varied portions of the physical organism.

Then, as the body does comprehend, does understand, does apply these truths, these conditions, these attributes within itself, the body of itself becomes its own best physician. And in the study of these conditions, whether related to the physical or mental body as we separate it for understanding spiritual attributes in the physical body, so may the body apply that necessary influence for healing in self, for keeping a proper balance, for maintaining a growing, developing mind, body, soul.

In keeping these, we would make these as suggestions for the body:

Know that Life in its manifestation is of that force called electrical, and in its vibrations as of positive and negative forces—in even the atoms or cells of the body—is builded by that which influences and, as has been shown, is of its own hereditary influence, by the active forces upon the vitamin forces.

Hence, when any necessary force is needed for creating this balance that may through emotion, through contact, through infection or the like at times become overactive or submerged in the numbers of the active forces between the positive and negative influences, it may be supplied by maintaining that balance through the lowest form of electrical vibration that may be created in the body; and, too, self may store within self's own body that which is natural in healing influence to others by laying on of hands, and by the stimulation of those vibrations necessary as may pass through any particular portion of another body that needs the creating of balance in that physical body.

Ready for questions.

(Q) Please explain more clearly how the body should go about a study of the low electrical vibratory forces.

(A) The low electrical vibratory forces are existent. They *are!* Or, as may be said, the lowest form of electrical vibration *is* the basis of life. The application of such vibrations to the body when it is fagged in mind, in physical endurance, will stimulate the necessary influences for the body to return to the abilities within self to carry on, or to create the life influence for self, or that it may measure out to others. Not necessarily that alone, but that known as the Radio-Active Appliance influence.

(Q) Please explain and give such advice regarding the glandular activity within this body that may be helpful in its development.

(A) Much might be given in this respect. The channels are weak through which this is being given in the present. These may be added, when the channels are cleared sufficient for better expression. But *this* for the body, [444] we are speaking of:

The glands (through experiences which the body is conscious of having passed) are being coordinated in more perfect manners than they have in a great period in the experience. And that the body has chosen through self's own will to make for a study of, and to open self for the acknowledging and experiencing of that which may be raised or lowered in vibration throughout the body, makes for not only a soul advancement but greater abilities in the mental equipment and the mental abilities and scope of activity of this body. 444-2

Final Choices

The above reading offers a glimpse of the holistic nature of the body as a unified energy field comprised of spiritual, mental, and physical forces. When the body's electrical vibrations become disturbed, they can be rebalanced through various means, including the Radio-Active Appliance. Maintaining the vibrational integrity of the body is one of the main functions of sleep. Unfortunately, Thomas Edison had no idea of this connection despite his knowledge of electricity. If he had, Edison might not have casually dismissed sleep as unnecessary. Instead, he would have understood Cayce's explanation that the body needs the rest provided by sufficient sleep to restore its energies to the optimum.

Perhaps the information presented in these pages has

given you a better understanding of sleep and its importance. It may be that you have also come to a deeper
regard for yourself as an individual, a soul in the image
of the Creator. If so, you may feel a greater sense of
responsibility about who and what you are and about
your purpose in life. Cayce asked an engineer if he were
living a purposeful life and then added:

> This is not a questioning of you. The question is in
> self! For each soul gives account for the deeds done
> in the body. Each soul gives account of the deeds
> done in the body!
> To whom do they account? The divine within their
> own selves. 3400-1

The questioning is always within yourself—and the
answers with them. If you sense any questioning at the
edge of your mind, perhaps it will nudge you to work
with some of the ideas discussed in this book. We are all
works in progress; and each of us has a purpose. Realizing your purpose—spiritually, mentally, physically—will
not only brighten your days, it will also give a tremendous boost to the quality of your slumber at night. You
will begin to sleep like a baby. And you deserve a good
night's sleep—just as you deserve pleasant dreams.

References and Recommended Reading

Alimaras, Peter, Ph.D. *How to Change Your Mind: Using Modern Psychological Methods and the Wisdom of Edgar Cayce*. Virginia Beach, Va.: A.R.E. Press, 1997.

Allen, James. *As a Man Thinketh*. Marina del Rey, Cal.: DeVorss & Company, Undated.

Bloomfield, Harold H., M.D. *Healing Anxiety with Herbs*. New York, N.Y.: HarperCollins Publishers, 1998.

Chopra, Deepak, M.D. *Ageless Body, Timeless Mind: The Quantum Alternative to Growing Old*. New York, N.Y.: Harmony Books, 1993.

———. *Quantum Healing: Exploring the Frontiers of Mind/Body Medicine*. New York, N.Y.: Bantam Books, 1990.

———. *Restful Sleep: The Complete Mind-Body Program for Overcoming Insomnia*. New York, N.Y.: Harmony Books, 1994.

Coren, Stanley. *Sleep Thieves: An Eye-Opening Exploration into the Science and Mysteries of Sleep*. New York, N.Y.: The Free Press, 1996.

Courtenay, Anthea. *Natural Sleep: How to Beat Insomnia Without Drugs*. Wellingborough, Northhamptonshire, England: Thorsons Publishing Group, 1988.

Cousins, Norman. *Anatomy of an Illness as Perceived by the Patient*. New York, N.Y.: W.W. Norton & Company, 1979.

Gabbay, Simone, RNCP *Nourishing the Body Temple*. Virginia Beach, Va.: A.R.E. Press, 1999.

Gnap, John J., M.D., with Nancy Flaster. *Easy Sleep*. New York, N.Y.: Stein and Day, 1978.

Goldberg, Philip, and Daniel Kaufman. *Everybody's Guide to Natural Sleep: A Drug-Free Approach to Overcoming Insomnia and Other Sleep Disorders*. Los Angeles, Cal.: Jeremy P. Tarcher, 1990.

———. *Natural Sleep (How to Get Your Share)*. Emmaus, Pa.: Rodale Press, 1978.

Graedon, Joe, and Teresa Graedon, Ph.D. *The People's Pharmacy Guide to Home and Herbal Remedies*. New York, N.Y.: St. Martin's Press, 1999.

Hauri, Peter, Ph.D., and Shirley Linde, Ph.D. *No More Sleepless Nights*. New York, N.Y.: John Wiley & Sons, 1990.

Ingalese, Richard. *The History and Power of the Mind*. North Hollywood, Cal.: Newcastle Publishing Co., 1976.

Irion, J. Everett. *Why Do We Dream?* Virginia Beach, Va.: A.R.E. Press, 1990.

Irion, J. Everett. *Vibrations*. Virginia Beach, Va.: A.R.E. Press, 1979.

Ouspensky, P.D. *A New Model of the Universe*. New York, N.Y.: Vintage Books, 1971.

Perl, James, Ph.D. *Sleep Right in Five Nights: A Clear and Effective Guide for Conquering Insomnia*. New York, N.Y.: William Morrow and Company, 1993.

Puryear, Herbert B., Ph.D. *Reflections on the Path*. Virginia Beach, Va.: A.R.E. Press, 1979.

Puryear, Herbert B., Ph.D., and Mark Thurston, Ph.D. *Meditation and the Mind of Man*. Virginia Beach, Va.: A.R.E. Press, 1975.

Reed, Henry. *Edgar Cayce on Mysteries of the Mind*. New York, N.Y.: Warner Books, 1989.

Reilly, Harold J., and Ruth Hagy Brod. *The Edgar Cayce Handbook for Health Through Drugless Therapy*. Virginia Beach, Va.: A.R.E. Press, 1975.

Ritchie, George G., with Elizabeth Sherrill. *Return from Tomorrow*. Waco, Tex.: Chosen Books, 1978.

Robertson, Jon. *The Golden Thread of Oneness*. Virginia Beach, Va.: A.R.E. Press, 1997.

Schwartz, Alice Kuhn, and Norma S. Aaron. *Somniquest: The 5 Types of Sleeplessness and How to Overcome Them*. New York, N.Y.: Harmony Books, 1979.

Sechrist, Elsie. *Meditation—Gateway to Light*. Virginia Beach, Va.: A.R.E. Press, 1964.

Smith, Robert C. *Attitude and Your Life! A Spiritually Based Action Plan for Self-Transformation*. Virginia Beach, Va.: A.R.E. Press, 1998.

Weil, Andrew, M.D. *Spontaneous Healing: How to Discover and Enhance Your Body's Natural Ability to Maintain and Heal Itself*. New York, N.Y.: Alfred A. Knopf, 1995.

Resources

American College of Sports Medicine
P.O. Box 1440
Indianapolis, IN 46206
317-637-9200
Fax: 317-634-7817
Internet: http://www.acsm.org

American Physical Therapy Association
111 North Fairfax St.
Alexandria, VA 22314-1488
800-999-2782
Fax: 703-706-3396
Internet: www.apta.org

American Sleep Apnea Association
1424 K Street NW, Suite 302
Washington, DC 20005
202-293-3650
Fax: 202-293-3656
E-mail: asaa@sleepapnea.org
Internet: http://www.sleepapnea.org

Better Sleep Council
333 Commerce Street
Alexandria, VA 22314
703-683-8371
Fax: 703-683-4503
Internet: http://www.bettersleep.org

Narcolepsy Network
10921 Reed Hartman Highway
Cincinnati, OH 45242
513-891-3522
Fax: 513-891-3836
E-mail: narnet@aol.com
Internet: http://www.websciences.org/narnet

National Institute on Aging Information Center
P.O. Box 8057
Gaithersburg, MD 20898-8057
800-222-2225
Internet: www.nih.gov/nia

National Sleep Foundation
1522 K Street NW, Suite 500
Washington, DC 20005
Fax: 202-347-3472.
Internet: http://www.websciences.org/nsf/

Restless Legs Syndrome Foundation, Inc.
819 Second Street SW
Rochester, MN 55902-2985
507-287-6465
Fax: 507-287-6312
E-mail: RLSFoundation@rls.org
Internet: http://www.rls.org

Sleep Research Society
1610-14th Street NW, Suite 300
Rochester, MN 55901
507-287-6006
Fax: 507-287-6008
Internet: http://www.srssleep.org

Wake Up America
701 Welch Road, Suite 2226
Palo Alto, CA 94304
650-725-6484
Fax: 650-725-7341
Internet: http://www.stanford.edu/~dement/wua.html

Cayce-Related Devices and Products:

Baar Products, Inc.
  P.O. Box 60
  Downingtown, PA 19335
  800-269-2502
  E-mail: bbaar@baar.com
  Internet: http://www.baar.com

Index

A.R.E. PRESS

The A.R.E. Press publishes quality books, videos, and audiotapes meant to improve the quality of our readers' lives—personally, professionally, and spiritually. We hope our products support your endeavors to realize your career potential, to enhance your relationships, to improve your health, and to encourage you to make the changes necessary to live a loving, joyful, and fulfilling life.

For more information or to receive a free catalog, call:

1-800-723-1112

Or write:

A.R.E. Press
215 67th Street
Virginia Beach, VA 23451-2061

DISCOVER HOW THE EDGAR CAYCE MATERIAL CAN HELP YOU!

The Association for Research and Enlightenment, Inc. (A.R.E.®), was founded in 1931 by Edgar Cayce. Its international headquarters are in Virginia Beach, Virginia, where thousands of visitors come year round. Many more are helped and inspired by A.R.E.'s local activities in their own hometowns or by contact via mail (and now the Internet!) with A.R.E. headquarters.

People from all walks of life, all around the world, have discovered meaningful and life-transforming insights in the A.R.E. programs and materials, which focus on such areas as personal spirituality, holistic health, dreams, family life, finding your best vocation, reincarnation, ESP, meditation, and soul growth in small-group settings. Call us today on our toll-free number:

1-800-333-4499

or

Explore our electronic visitors center on the Internet: **http://www.edgarcayce.org.**

We'll be happy to tell you more about how the work of the A.R.E. can help you!

A.R.E.
215 67th Street
Virginia Beach, VA 23451-2061